OUTSMART
ENDOMETRIOSIS

Relieve Your Symptoms
and Get Your Career
Back on Track

DR. JESSICA DRUMMOND

ISBN: 978-19-5-036750-4

Published by

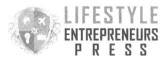
LIFESTYLE ENTREPRENEURS PRESS

If you are interested in publishing through Lifestyle Entrepreneurs Press, write to: *Publishing@LifestyleEntrepreneursPress.com*

Publications or foreign rights acquisition of our catalog books. Learn More: *www.LifestyleEntrepreneursPress.com*

Printed in the USA

Advance Praise

"Have you ever had a medical professional downplay or dismiss your symptoms? Endometriosis can be an extremely painful, frustrating, and lonely condition. But in *Outsmart Endometriosis*, you have an ally to help you get answers, solutions, and hope. While working with a skilled surgeon can bring incredible relief for some women, what often gets left out of the endometriosis treatment plan is nutrition and lifestyle therapy. These are the steps that everyone with endometriosis can make daily to move towards a better state of health. Dr. Jessica Drummond, a skilled physical therapist and nutritionist with decades of clinical experience in supporting women with endometriosis provides you with an integrative approach to endometriosis that teaches you to tailor it to meet your body's needs. This isn't about food being the enemy, this is about understanding how food affects your condition.

As a women's health naturopathic physician I have seen tremendous outcomes using this approach, and have witnessed patient after patient take back their health and do the things their doctors said could never be done, like living pain free.

You have the power to heal and *Outsmart Endometriosis* will show you how."

—Dr. Jolene Brighten, best-selling author,
Beyond the Pill

"As the author of *Heal Pelvic Pain* and the co-author of *Beating Endo: How to Reclaim your life with Endometriosis*, and having seen thousands of patients with Endo, I know how challenging it can be to write a clear and comprehensive book that addresses the many aspects to healing and recovery. Jessica's book does just that! Congrats Jessica!"

—Amy Stein, Owner of Beyond Basics Physical Therapy and co-author of *Beating Endo*

"*Outsmart Endometriosis* is informative and exceptionally uplifting. This book is a game-changer and is a must-read for anyone that suffers from endo, endo related symptoms or is a support system for someone with endo. Author, Dr. Jessica Drummond guides readers down a path that allows for incredible healing from the root cause. Her powerful integrative approach to endometriosis should be an essential part of every treatment plan.

Outsmart Endometriosis is a comprehensive and thorough resource that will educate you and empower you. The book gives readers a roadmap to navigate the nuances of this complex and invisible disease — and provides nutritional strategies and lifestyle changes to regain your health. Dr. Drummond outlines vital information in a way that is relatable and simple to integrate into daily life. As a highly educated nutritionist, seasoned pelvic physical therapist and sought after expert in women's and pelvic health conditions she shares her extensive knowledge in this book. She provides readers with the crucial tools needed to create an individual plan that can truly help relieve your endometriosis symptoms so you can take control of your life.

As an endometriosis patient myself who has had life-changing results, fine-tuning my own highly individualized plan with Dr. Drummond — I can speak first hand to the power of her integrative approach. I highly recommend Dr. Jessica Drummond and her book *Outsmart Endometriosis*. I know the book's impact will reach far and wide. It will change your life."

– Katie Bormaster

"I have been waiting for a book like this. This book is a must have! While you read this, you will feel the author, Jessica's, heart and brain. She intertwines herself and her past struggles so it is easy to feel a connection to her passion in this book. As someone with Endometriosis I felt like there was a supportive voice throughout this book powering me through my journey forward. This book is full of information that will help anyone in any stage of their endometriosis, even if they suspect the diagnosis. The medical talk is written in a way that makes it easy to understand. The recipes are made with real foods that you can easily find, and are delicious! The advice is clear and evidence based. You will be so glad that you have this book and will refer back to it over and over. Jessica Drummond is a leader in the Women's Health Industry and reading this book it is clear why. I cannot recommend this book more. It can help you, or someone that you know. You will NOT be disappointed!"

– Amy Velasquez Rempel

*For my patients. Your bravery inspires me every day
to innovate and challenge the status quo.
The world needs you!*

Contents

Foreword

I met Jessica Drummond in 2013 and she has been instrumental in my healing journey, where I not only healed from endometriosis, but got pregnant and gave birth in December 2016 to my dear twin boys.

Just so you know where I am coming from, I personally was first diagnosed with endometriosis back in 2011. Initially, I had no clue what that meant for me. Having grown up in France, I thought and believed that doctors held the cure for any disease. I believed that the surgery I was recommended to confirm endometriosis would help remove it and that the hormonal pills and injections I was later prescribed would remove whatever was left of it.

But it wasn't like that. As many of you probably know.

If you have endometriosis, you probably know already that reducing the impact of endometriosis on your life and healing from it is not that easy. You might have been on the pill for most of your life. You might have had several surgeries already – knowing that the last one is probably not the last one! You might have had relationships break over your condition because the people around you didn't understand how you could have so much pain. Or you might have had doctors tell you that you needed to have your whole uterus removed, or that you will never get pregnant. There are so many things I lived through and heard that you probably have too.

At the time though, I didn't know that you could really heal from endometriosis. It's not easy, but it is possible. You need the right guidance! And this is where Jessica's amazing book comes in.

I personally went from being in great physical pain and emotional distress almost daily to feeling a lot more like my old self within six months of implementing most of the changes she recommends.

I was lucky enough to be able to take some time off work to embark on a journey of discovery for healing – mind, body and soul. Following my diagnosis of endometriosis in 2011, I had a burnout in 2013. I was overworked, so clearly that didn't help. Yet it was a chance for me to take some time off. Even as I discovered more tools and resources to help myself and better understand what was working for my body and what was not, the pain had not completely left me within a year of starting that work.

I was looking for a proven holistic approach that was both rooted in science and experience, and would help me to create more impact in my healing journey. That's when I discovered Jessica Drummond and her work on pelvic pain. I enrolled into her certification course and was truly amazed at the level of research she had done into what was working in terms of healing pelvic pain and, more specifically, endometriosis.

Thanks to me implementing what she taught, I was able to reduce my pain even further to the point where it was almost non-existent. The pain would only come back when I was overstressed, which when you understand the hormonal cascade, you know is a clear side effect. I was also able to optimize my fertility and get pregnant with twins on my first intracytoplasmic sperm injection (ICSI) trial. We implanted two fertilized embryos, and two healthy children were born from it.

Now, if you look at the statistics, you will see that endometriosis is already the cause for infertility in twenty-five to thirty-five percent of women worldwide. Out of the women who have endometriosis, fifty percent of them will have trouble getting pregnant. Add on top azoospermia (which my husband had) and your likelihood of getting pregnant on the first trial of ICSI and giving birth to all the implanted embryos reduces even further.

But thanks to the recommendations and support from Jessica, this was made possible.

Even without talking about fertility, looking into the solutions that Jessica presents will make you feel more at peace with your own body. Sometimes when you are in a great deal of pain you might feel like your body is failing you. Through this work, you will understand that this is in fact the opposite. As you get more in tune with what is creating these levels of pain (both physical and emotional), you will move to a place where you feel more comfortable choosing what is working and what is not.

I strongly believe when you want to heal from endometriosis, you need to make a commitment to yourself and become the authority in your health journey. You are the person that knows you and your body best. So you should be the person deciding what you are going to do.

From that perspective, I recommend that you pick up Jessica's book. You will feel empowered to create a holistic plan of action for your healing journey. As soon as you start to see results in the right direction, you will feel even more empowered to implement the solutions she teaches you.

This is both my personal recommendation as an ex-endometriosis sufferer and my professional recommendation as a certified women's health and nutrition coach.

To another right step in your healing journey,

Audrey Sourroubille Arnold
Certified Women's Health and Nutrition Coach
at Lotus Power Health

CHAPTER 1

You Are the Expert at Powering through Pain

Your boss, colleagues, even your family and friends might not believe that your pain is real. But I believe you. I have had the honor of supporting thousands of people through their endometriosis healing journeys, and I know that you're doing the very best you can. While I have never been diagnosed with endometriosis, I have experienced very intense pelvic pain and four years of an invisible illness that sidelined me from doing the work I loved in women's health.

I was in my early thirties when I got really sick. I felt like my body – and many days my mind – was failing me, just when I was hitting my stride in my career.

You're probably like me. You *want* to show up for your classes, important meetings, clients, patients, performances, and presentations. You have goals. You're smart, capable, and have been working behind the scenes to keep your pain, fatigue, anxiety, and other symptoms under wraps as best as you can. But sometimes you get tired. You're tired of powering through. You're exhausted from years of showing up for tests, presentations, performances, deadlines, and meetings while breathing through intense pain, constant fatigue, and chronic anxiety. This is all while taking handfuls of medications, most of which didn't help, or if they did, didn't last.

Seventy-five percent of women with endometriosis feel that they have not reached their life potential because of this disease (Tu, et al., 2019). It is financially stressful and impacts your ability to show up for important events, say "yes" to big opportunities, and be there even when work is stressful. You want to learn how to optimize your energy, reduce your pain, and manage your symptoms so you can reach your potential at school, at work, and in life.

You're frustrated by going from doctor to doctor and having them tell you things like, "It's normal to have pain with your periods." "Lots of women have IBS, it's probably nothing." "Just have a glass of wine before sex, relax, and you'll be fine." "I don't see anything wrong with you." And much, much worse.

You're tired of your teachers, school nurses, colleagues, and employers thinking that you're exaggerating or just trying to get out of a test, presentation, or high-stress meeting. You spend all night taking your meds, using the heat and ice packs, and worrying about how you are going to be able to show up – because you want to show up. You enjoy your work. You have friends there. You want to use your talents to help your students, patients, and readers. You want a successful career. You deserve a successful career.

By now, you might have already downshifted. Maybe you slowed down your university or graduate program, have taken extended leave, gone part time, or shifted to freelance work. You've had to adjust in order to be able to set your own hours, work around your fatigue, and not have to be embarrassed on the days your body just can't be at that important meeting.

You're Not Alone

You're not alone. There are 176 million people in the world who have endometriosis and are powering through their pain and other symptoms too many days of every year. They are powering through just to show up – just like you. Endometriosis is a thief. It tries to rob you of your most productive years. It shows up and intensifies just as you're doing some of your most important work in school or your career.

Fortunately, I have had the opportunity to support thousands of women with endometriosis – lawyers, healthcare professionals, writers, teachers, actors, artists, and business women. I have seen how, with the right holistic approach to healing endometriosis, including a good professional team and personal support, these women were able to return to and progress in their careers. I have seen women go from being limited to very part-time work (or being sidelined from work completely) to enjoying and excelling at full-time, successful careers.

As you know, reducing your pain, fatigue, and other symptoms is well worth it, even if you never even go back to work. But it's even more important if you desire to have a productive career. Your desires are not frivolous. They are necessary. If you don't do the work that you're uniquely talented to do, who will? Sure, there are other teachers, writers, and lawyers, but none of them approach the work exactly the way that you do. None of them will have the exact same relationship as you do with your students, audiences, readers, patients, and clients. The world needs your insights, skills, and creativity.

You deserve to have financial stability and success, the pleasure of being productive, and relationships with colleagues that help you to grow. When you have a strategy and a plan that will reduce your overall endometriosis symptoms and support you to move through more challenging or stressful days, work becomes easier, the fear and feeling like a flake (even though you are *not*), the embarrassment and frustration fade. You're able to commit to bigger opportunities and get the career and financial rewards that your work deserves.

I want you to have the plan and path forward that has been successful for the patients in my practice that will enable you to feel healthier day-to-day, as well as navigate and grow your career successfully, even with this invisible disease. While there is no magic "cure" for endometriosis, there is a comprehensive approach that will significantly reduce or even fully relieve your symptoms, and give you control over managing any residual flares that happen from time to time in more stressful situations. It will be worth investing time to implement the steps in this book to relieve your symptoms, so you that you have energy and freedom from pain.

Unfortunately, not learning the essential information in this book can cost you your career. I have seen terrible results when the fear of taking the reins of recovery was too great to overcome. I have seen a skilled and committed nurse give up her career and be forced to sell her house and move back home with her unsupportive family. I have seen a brilliant business strategist power through her pain for about a year at a time but exhaust herself so much in the process that she had to quit and start her career over at least three times. Not having a clear path for healing and working can be devastating for your finances, career progress, and the life that you want to create.

To be clear, none of these devastating consequences were the fault of the women in my practice. Endometriosis is a terrible disease, and everyone who struggles with it is doing the best that they can. I want you to understand that there is a comprehensive path to healing that will support you to have a full life that includes meaningful work, even if you have a very severe case of endometriosis. The earlier that you step on this path of healing, the easier your journey will be.

I have seen this holistic approach work for the clients in my practice. I have had the honor of seeing Annabelle go from struggling through law school to passing the bar, getting a great first job, getting married, and getting pregnant within less than three years. I supported Jeanne's transition from working as a stressed out and struggling hospital-based physical therapist to getting her symptoms under control and opening her own practice to help other women overcome pelvic pain conditions. And Amanda, who is a very successful writer and producer. She only took freelance projects or short-term opportunities until she found this path of empowered healing, and now she's on a long-term project that has given her great success and helped her overcome her fear of committing to long-term team opportunities without worrying that she'll have to miss important meetings or deadlines. She no longer fears looking like a flake or losing her credibility with her colleagues.

I have worked with women in a wide variety of industries, including medicine, the arts, law, business, teaching, and everything in-between. If you're ready to gain control over your endometriosis symptoms and your career path during these important and highly productive years of your life, I am here to support you to be as successful as possible. Your success is a gift to every person that your work touches.

Let's begin the journey...

CHAPTER 2

Your Work Matters – Why You Need *All* of the Tools for Healing Your Endometriosis

What I want to share with you was originally born of my experience with my own chronic and debilitating illness, and how I brought what I learned from that experience back to my practice as a pelvic health physical therapist.

Endometriosis can feel like a mystery. In some ways, it is. We still don't know the specific cause of endometriosis, and it's not clear why some people have such severe symptoms, while others have mild ones, or even none at all. While we don't know the cause, we do know that every person who struggles with a chronic illness struggles with the day-to-day management of symptoms, and that has a direct impact on your life, work, and career goals.

That's a struggle I understand. You see, when I was in my early thirties, I began to experience a vague and slowly worsening decline in my health. I had insomnia, crushing fatigue, and was knocked down by chronic infections and viruses. My hormones went haywire, causing me to struggle with everything from hot flashes to intense anxiety, even panic attacks. I developed a driving phobia that haunts me to this day. My husband had to scoop me up off the floor lying next to my daughter's bed to take me to the emergency room twice for my severe pelvic pain. (There were other times when the pain was just as bad, but I didn't want to go to the hospital because I knew they couldn't do anything for me.) I experienced the frustration and sadness of infertility and miscarriage for four years. Day-to-day tasks like driving to work, caring for my patients, and playing with, feeding, and putting my daughter to sleep were impossible on my worst days.

When my mystery illness began, I was already a practicing women's health physical therapist and had worked in some of the top hospitals in the United States. Despite everything I learned and knew from my training and experience, and having access to top doctors and other health professionals, I suffered for four years before anyone had a clue what was wrong with me. I was dismissed by many doctors and told it was normal to be sick and tired when you have a young infant/toddler/child. I was told to take naps. I was told not to miss work. ("Just wear a mask if you're sick.") I was given antidepressants and sleeping medications and offered opioids. I went to psychotherapy and exercised intensely. But nothing helped.

Finally, after about four years of constant struggle, I found a physician who practiced functional medicine. She literally saved my life because of what she taught me about how to support my body to heal.

Until this illness completely knocked me down, I was just like you. I was high achieving! If I was sick, anxious, tired, or in pain, I took handfuls of ibuprofen, did some deep breathing, and showed up. I often came home and crashed, or hid in the bathroom until I could put on an "I'm fine" face. But I was always able to power though and show up eventually. In fact, the only time that I was forced to miss anything school or work-related for more than a few days was my senior year of high school. I was diagnosed with Epstein-Barr virus (aka "mono") and had to miss weeks of school. But I still slept, got up, did homework, and kept up with my classes. I graduated on time, and went on to college with the rest of my class.

What happened to me in my early thirties was a reactivation of the Epstein-Barr virus triggered by the birth of my first daughter that none of my doctors suspected, and I didn't even figure out for years. Thus, while I don't have endometriosis, I have experienced vague chronic illness and what it means to try to power through your schooling and work when you're battling feeling awful. Every day can feel like a struggle, and it's exhausting. Plus, I felt like a failure, which I was not used to and didn't take well. I was used to being able to appear "fine" in public most of the time. When I had to fully quit my job to heal, it was devastating. But I really had no choice. At that point, I had to focus on healing. Still, it was deeply unsettling and disorienting to feel so uncertain about what would come of my career, even my ability to work. I was scared.

I didn't immediately quit. For years I tried to keep up appearances. I felt like a flake.

You probably also know what it's like to feel like a flake – when you know that you're not! To have to miss important meetings, quit projects that you really want to do, because you just can't power through anymore. I completely understand.

When Pelvic Physical Therapy (Even after Surgery) Is Not Enough to Relieve the Pain of Endometriosis

By the time I got sick, I had worked with thousands of women with pelvic pain related to endometriosis. And I couldn't understand why some of them wouldn't get fully better even with good physical therapy. What I learned through my personal experience is that I was missing some tools to help them heal.

What taught me the most was working with thousands more women with endometriosis and the related pelvic pain and digestive, hormone, mood, and other symptoms that they experienced. I combined that personal and professional experience with going back to school to get a doctorate in clinical nutrition. Clinically, combining physical therapy with clinical nutrition, plus health coaching, lifestyle medicine, trauma informed psychotherapy, and often medication and surgery is the complete holistic toolbox you need to understand and get root-cause healing of your symptoms so you can get back to your work and your life!

The exciting news is that there is a systematic and inter-disciplinary approach that you can learn to gain power over your symptoms (not the other way around). Supporting you to "do it yourself" really is the goal of this book and of all of our programs at The Integrative Women's Health Institute. Ultimately, my goal is to help you learn daily self-healing strategies combined with support at work and home to manage your symptoms, show up for important days in your career, and laser focus on your nutrition, sleep, or other self-care. Plus, these strategies can empower you to navigate the complex healthcare system and find a team of healers to support your journey with education, coaching, and sometimes medication, physical therapy, and/or surgery.

The tools in this book are designed to be used every day, and as needed. A daily commitment to your health and a self-care practice, along with a team approach to healthcare *with* your professional team is how you can use this process to relieve your symptoms from the root causes. Once you have the tools to better manage your symptoms, you can shift your energy and attention back to growing your career and enjoying your life.

But first, I want to share a story with you. *A Tale of Two Patients*, if you will, that first demonstrated to me how the tools I learned to heal my own health could be powerful medicine for my patients with endometriosis.

In 2009, I worked with two different women around the same time who were both suspected to have endometriosis based on their symptoms. One, Jen, was a promising business student in Pennsylvania, and the other, Anna, had recently graduated from nursing school in North Carolina and was about two years into her first job.

Jen was knee-deep in school, working, and deepening her relationship with her fiancé. She was planning to get married, move, and start her new consulting job in New York City in about a year. But she was struggling to finish school because she had very severe pelvic pain every month and a lot of fatigue. Plus, she struggled with chronic yeast infections. So, for six months I supported her to clean up her diet, moderate her heavy exercise, build a mindfulness practice, have a non-negotiable bedtime, talk to her professors and her family, and ask for a lot of help. In the meantime, she met with a highly skilled and experienced endometriosis surgeon who recommended excision surgery. For six months she diligently followed the plan, got support from her family and professors, and got her body ready for surgery. She still had a lot of pain but had a lot of tools to manage and better predict her pain.

Her surgery was successful. She then spent another eighteen months or so recovering, integrating her daily self-care practice, and finishing her MBA. She got married, moved, and started her job. The entire time she continued to eat well, take her supplements, see her pelvic physical therapist, work with a therapist to address her challenges with sexual intimacy with her new husband, and was patient with her surgical recovery. She prioritized rest and avoided drinking alcohol or staying out too late with her friends and colleagues, even while attending the many weddings she was invited to that year. She very much enjoyed her life, and concurrently, she learned and appreciated her need to pace herself. With surprise and joy, less than two years after her surgery, she got pregnant with her first baby on her first attempt, without any need for medical assistance, and had a healthy baby boy.

In contrast, Anna resisted reducing her schedule, did not prioritize her sleep, did not seek counseling, and did not have a supportive family. She was under a lot of financial pressure, including significant student loans and a home mortgage.

She was very afraid to slow down. She felt paralyzed by her financial stressors, and was determined not to "look weak" in front of her family, friends, and colleagues. She was terrified of asking for help due to her challenging and, at times, traumatic relationship with her family. She adopted their beliefs that she wasn't really that sick, that she was exaggerating, and that she "should" be able to handle this on her own. I understood and empathized with her feelings of being trapped. I was certainly scared when I had to quit my job and move to a small house in a city I didn't love in order to commit to my healing. None of what she was going to have to do would be easy. When you have a mortgage, student loans, a job with crazy hours that you don't feel like you can quit, and an unsupportive family, the stress is overwhelming.

And yet, what I and many of my patients committed to doing was to prioritize this kind of healing approach, no matter what. No matter how weak we would appear to others. Even when it meant selling a house, moving across the country, and leaning on friends when family wasn't helpful. This isn't always an easy journey, but it's an important one if you want to reach your health, career, and life goals.

Anna did the best she could with the cards she was given. It can feel impossibly difficult to overcome the beliefs and lack of support of your family of origin. I don't blame her at all for submitting to her fear. We all do that sometimes.

Ultimately, Anna ended up having surgery performed by her local gynecologist. But she was not able to adequately prepare for the surgery with good nutrition, lifestyle changes, medicine, and physical therapy. The surgery was not successful. She struggled to recover and ended up with some very severe complications. She has since had to sell her house, go on disability, and move back in with her family anyway. She is now working with a great local team, including a functional medicine physician, a nutritionist and health coach who was trained at the institute I founded, and a skilled pelvic health physical therapist. It took hitting rock bottom for her to overcome her fear and prioritize her healing. She was left with no other option. She's in good hands now, and she has decided to be the leader in her healing journey – committing to her daily practice of self-care, boundary setting, and reaching out for support. She eventually recovered enough to get back to nursing. But the road was long, and she required additional surgery before she was able to even take some baby steps back to part-time work.

The contrast of having worked with both of these women at nearly the same time was so impactful to me that it changed the course of my career. Of course, there is always the risk that even if you follow all of the recommendations in this book and see the top physical therapists, endometriosis physicians, and surgeons in the world, you could still end up with significant symptoms or complications. That is the risk that we all have to take. There are no guarantees in life. But after working with thousands of people with endometriosis over the last two decades, I have had the opportunity to witness many wonderful stories of healing when they fully commit to their health for a few months in the short term. This leads them to have long-term, root-cause healing that makes it much easier to move forward with satisfying careers and lives that are no longer limited by endometriosis. As you learn these tools, you will also experience more and more resilience in your health in general. The sooner you can begin the better.

There is unfortunately not a one-size-fits-all "Endo Diet." If there were, this would be a much easier plan to teach and a much easier book to write. Fortunately, there is a systematic approach, a step-by-step plan that will help you to figure out the right endometriosis nutrition and lifestyle medicine plan for you, so that you can get your health back and your symptoms under control. With power over your endometriosis symptoms, you'll be able to devote your energy to having a great career and life!

In the next chapter, you'll learn all about the steps of your healing plan. I love to support my clients and patients in working though this plan with at least one or two additional supportive people. In many cases, the person who has endometriosis is not the only one struggling. Your partner, close friends, or family members may be frustrated by the fact that they don't know what to do to help you. They hate to see you in pain, anxious, or exhausted. Being able to give them specific recipes to cook for you, or strategies to do with you, like meditation or breathing exercises, can feel empowering for you and those who care about you.

In fact, many of my patients have partners or friends who became much better cooks and dedicated themselves to learning how to cook the anti-inflammatory, nourishing foods that are so supportive of endometriosis healing. When the people in your life take the time and effort to learn to cook to support your healing, they get healthier and have more energy as well, and they feel empowered as a part of your healing team. Let the people who love you help. You may be surprised at how much it helps them to have something concrete that they can do to help you. They also want to see you healthy and showing up with energy in your work and life. When you commit to your own healing, some of these same strategies that you use to address your endometriosis symptoms will help your husband with headaches, your daughter with asthma, and your mom with diabetes. As you commit to your health with a concrete plan, you will inspire and help others to do the same.

"The rising tide lifts all the boats."
—John F. Kennedy

CHAPTER 3

Healing Endometriosis – The Roadmap

Beginning in the next chapter, you will learn the details of exactly how to follow a systematic approach to healing your endometriosis. This process is specifically designed to reduce your endometriosis symptoms and give you the energy and focus to get your attention back to your career, so that you can have success and the life that you deserve.

In just two short years I went from being debilitated by my symptoms – not able to even get out of bed some mornings to drive my four-year-old to school – to getting back to full-time work. I have since been able to build a business that today serves thousands of women's health practitioners and hundreds of thousands of people with pelvic pain to heal in more than sixty countries around the world. However, even today – more than a decade later – I still personally use all of the tools in this book to maintain and enhance my health. It's a process of deciding each day to prioritize my health by what I choose to eat, how I choose to move, setting and keeping my boundaries in my work and relationships, and knowing when to rest and ask for help. Soon, you will have these tools and this power in your hands.

First, you'll learn whether or not you actually have endometriosis by getting a clear diagnosis. Ultimately, endometriosis is a surgical diagnosis. But your healthcare team can have a strong suspicion and that is enough to recommend you start treatment without doing surgery immediately. Most physicians who are experienced with endometriosis can decide based on symptoms, some imaging, and lab tests, whether or not someone is *likely* to have endometriosis. Even if you later find out that you don't have endometriosis based on a skilled and experienced surgical diagnosis, if you follow the plan in this book, you will still likely improve your symptoms.

Many symptoms of chronic pain, fatigue, digestive issues, and mood challenges have common root causes, such as inflammation, stress, digestive or immune system dysfunction, gut microbiome dysbiosis, or nutrient deficiencies. By addressing all of these symptom drivers with this nutrition and lifestyle approach, you can help reduce your symptoms, even if you aren't ever officially diagnosed with endometriosis by laproscopy. Even those with an official endometriosis diagnosis often have other health challenges that may actually be driving the symptoms or making the endometriosis symptoms worse.

Then, in Chapter 5, you'll learn that not all of your symptoms are directly caused by endometriosis. Endometriosis often presents with a wide variety of comorbidities from depression to autoimmune disease to constipation to other chronic pain conditions like fibromyalgia. When you use the nutrition and lifestyle medicine strategies in this book, you'll be able to improve all of your symptoms, even if some of them are actually being caused by other conditions that commonly occur with endometriosis. When you have a clear plan to support the health of all of your systems, especially your digestive, immune, nervous, and musculoskeletal systems, your focus will be on optimizing your complete physical health. Then you can let go of chasing symptoms with short-term options that don't get to the root of the problem.

Next, you'll learn strategies to help you create a plan for explaining your condition to your employer and managing your day-to-day energy. Your goal through treatment will be to focus your energy on healing as much as possible, while also keeping your job, if necessary. Concurrently, you'll create a vision for how you'd like your career to grow once you have reduced or resolved your symptoms, and you have the time, attention, and energy you need to focus on advancing your career. Even once you've dramatically improved your endometriosis symptoms and you're well along the healing journey, you'll still have to maintain your healing nutrition, stress management, movement, and mindset approach to keep you at the top of your game! You will have to learn to integrate time for rest and recovery, and know when and how to push through and work harder and longer when important or exciting opportunities arise.

Once you have a clear plan for maintaining your career, in Chapter 7 you'll learn the step-by-step process for coming up with your unique best nutrition plan for healing. There's no one-size-fits-all "Endo Diet" for everyone. But there is a specific nutrition plan that you'll learn will be foundational for *your* healing and long-term health. Over time you'll build resilience and your nutrition plan will likely become more flexible. But in the short term, you'll need to be diligent about the anti-inflammatory, nutrient-dense nutrition plan that's personalized to your body's healing needs to get the most out of all of your other therapies.

Once your nutrition plan is clarified, you'll learn to use supplements to support digestion, lower inflammation, and manage symptom flares. While you can't exercise, medicate, or supplement your way out of a poor diet, adding personalized, targeted supplementation can absolutely accelerate your healing. As you better understand how specific supplements are helpful, you'll be able to use them when you become more resilient and are working more intensely to enhance your work performance. A personalized supplement plan can also give you some extra support when you have busy or more stressful work days.

In Chapter 9, you'll learn how your own brain chemistry and mindset are surprisingly powerful tools for pain relief, relieving depression and anxiety, improving fatigue and brain focus, and helping you to sleep. Learn to use nutrition, supplementation, and lifestyle strategies like yoga, vagus nerve toning, breathing exercises, and more to optimize your brain health. While none of your symptoms are "in your head," pain signaling does originate in the brain. When you learn to relieve your nervous system inflammation and properly nourish your brain, your brain will no longer send so many danger signals, including pain, anxiety, and fatigue.

Finally, you'll learn how to build a team. When you step into the leadership role in your healing team, you can get the help you need to get support and education for interdisciplinary root cause healing. You'll learn how to choose great surgeons, physicians, physical therapists, psychologists, nutritionists, coaches and more to give you the therapies, education, and tools that you need to accelerate the pace of your healing, and manage symptom flares at any time.

As you read through this book, read the chapters in order because the process builds on itself. You may not complete the steps in order during your personal healing journey, but this holistic approach will be easier to understand when read in order. Also, keep a journal handy and jot down questions that come up for you along the way. Some parts of this process, especially some of the physiology, science, lab testing, and supplement details can get a bit complex and can bring up questions of how you should use these recommendations in your unique circumstances. If you write down questions as you read, you can bring them to your professional healing team who can answer your questions in the specific context of your unique physiology, disease process, resources, and other factors.

CHAPTER 4

Do I Really Have Endometriosis?

Endometriosis is challenging to diagnose and can be misdiagnosed. Before you take the steps in the coming chapters to relieve your symptoms, let's consider whether or not you likely are truly dealing with endometriosis. (Note: If you have some of these symptoms but not a clear endometriosis diagnosis, many of the nutrition, lifestyle medicine, and self-care tools that you'll learn in this book will still be helpful for your healing journey.)

What is Endometriosis?

Endometriosis is a disease in which tissue similar to (but not exactly the same as) the tissue that normally lines the inside of your uterus, called the endometrium, grows in lesions outside of your uterus. These lesions are most commonly present in the abdominopelvic cavity, such as on the pelvic organs or bowel. But the endometrial-like tissue and lesions can be found far from the pelvic organs, such as on the lungs. The lesions can become inflamed, grow, and/ or spread, and can contribute to adhesions or the development of scar tissue.

Diagnosing Endometriosis

Endometriosis is a challenging diagnosis because while symptoms, lab data, and imaging can be helpful, ultimately endometriosis can only be confirmed or ruled out with a skilled laparoscopic surgical assessment. Laparoscopy is a surgical procedure used to examine the abdominal and pelvic organs. It's a low-risk, minimally invasive procedure using small cameras to observe the tissues and perform surgery requiring only small incisions. We'll discuss this in more detail later, and it does not mean that every woman with endometriosis must have surgery, but I strongly suggest that you get a surgeon on your healing team who is highly skilled in endometriosis excision surgery. In fact, if at all possible, find a surgeon who specializes in only endometriosis or at least endometriosis and other similar diagnoses.

Before seeking surgical diagnosis, you and your healing team will consider other things to decide whether or not you likely have endometriosis. There are pelvic pain conditions that are not endometriosis, and while some of the treatment is similar, it's not always the same. Thus, ideally, you want to be sure that you're at least very likely dealing with endometriosis.

Common Endometriosis Symptoms

The first step to getting a clear diagnosis (or not) of endometriosis is to consider the clinical picture. How those with endometriosis experience the disease varies. The symptoms include bleeding between periods, heavy bleeding, painful periods (dysmenorrhea), pelvic pain that is not consistent with the menstrual cycle (especially in teenagers), painful intercourse (dyspareunia), painful defecation (dyschezia), and painful urination (dysuria) (Parasar, Ozcan & Terry, 2017).

These symptoms can present even before or in very early puberty, especially digestive symptoms, abdominal pain, and pelvic pain when girls are approximately eight through thirteen. Plus, in some cases endometriosis is asymptomatic (Parasar, Ozcan & Terry, 2017). In these cases, endometriosis is "silent" without any obvious symptoms of pain, fatigue, menstrual cycle issues, or other symptoms commonly associated with endometriosis. For some people, endometriosis is only suspected when there is a struggle with infertility.

Most people with endometriosis do present with symptoms, but most have normal physical gynecologic exams (Parasar, Ozcan & Terry, 2017). Sometimes a gynecologist will find pelvic tenderness (especially of the posterior fornix, the deep space in the back of the vagina near the cervix) during their exam. Other causes of pelvic pain such as pelvic adhesions, gastrointestinal issues, or bladder pain symptoms can occur with endometriosis, or might be causing the pain, even if no endometriosis lesions are present.

Do Lab Tests or Imaging Confirm a Diagnosis of Endometriosis?

Unfortunately, no. While a lot of research has focused on finding a gold standard blood, urine, stool, or other lab test, no simple or reliable biomarkers of endometriosis have been found for early noninvasive or semi-invasive diagnosis of this disease (Parasar, Ozcan & Terry, 2017). Many studies have evaluated the diagnostic usefulness of biomarkers for endometriosis (Vodolazkaia, et al., 2012). But at this point, there are no reliable recommended biomarkers in endometrial tissue or menstrual or uterine fluids, or immunologic markers in blood or urine that have been found clinically useful to diagnose endometriosis.

There are a number of biomarkers that when taken together or individually can give doctors more information about each person's case of endometriosis. These include:

- inflammatory markers (such as IL-1, TNF-α, CRP, etc.)
- hormones and their receptors
- growth factors (such as insulin-like growth factor (IGF))
- cell adhesion and extracellular matrix molecules
- markers of angiogenesis, apoptosis, and cell cycle control
- stem cell markers
- genetic markers
- tissue remodeling markers (such as matrix metallopro-teinase-2 (MMP-2) and urokinase)

Thus, it's useful to talk with your doctor and other healthcare professionals to see if you have any elevated inflammatory markers, signs of inflammation, genetic markers that are common to endometriosis, or other laboratory signs that are common in people with endometriosis. Talk with your endometriosis specialist to learn more about the biomarkers they most commonly consider in their assessment and if any of these markers makes sense to test in the context of your history. Testing is usually only relevant in the context of a clinical history and physical exam.

Pelvic ultrasounds can help to clarify the diagnosis if a woman has fibroids, ovarian cysts, or endometriomas (Parasar,

Ozcan & Terry, 2017). Sometimes more than one of these issues can be present in the same person. Transvaginal ultrasound is another noninvasive test that uses sound waves to visualize and assess the endometrium and uterine cavity. Transvaginal ultrasounds can detect ovarian endometriotic cysts. But if nothing is seen on the pelvic or transvaginal ultrasounds, peritoneal endometriosis, endometriosis-associated adhesions, and deep infiltrating endometriosis cannot be ruled out. Occasionally, other imaging such as magnetic resonance imaging (MRI) and computed tomography (CT) scans can give more detail about the pelvic masses. Talking to your doctor will help you to decide if imaging studies may help you learn more about what could be causing your symptoms. Experts disagree about the usefulness of imaging to improve the ease of diagnosis of endometriosis.

Where Does Endometriosis Occur?

Endometriosis can exist in one location or a variety of locations. The lesions can be superficial or deep and infiltrating into the tissues they invaded. For example, endometriosis lesions can be found on the muscles of the uterus, in the walls of the fallopian tubes, in the lesser pelvis – including the ovaries, and on the Pouch of Douglas, which is located between the rectum and the uterus. Endometriosis lesions can also be located on the uterosacral ligaments, the bowel, bladder, and in rarer cases the lungs and other organs including the diaphragm, liver, pancreas, and gallbladder. Nasal endometriosis has even been identified in rare cases (Mignemi, et al., 2012).

Skilled Endometriosis Excision Surgery Is the Gold Standard for Endometriosis Diagnosis

The gold standard for confirming a diagnosis of endometriosis is laparoscopic inspection with histologic confirmation after biopsy (Kennedy, et al., 2005). Endometriotic lesions are visualized by the use of laparoscope, ideally by a skilled surgeon who specializes in working with patients with endometriosis. It's also important to be aware that the extent of the disease (how many lesions, where they are located, etc.) does not correlate well with how symptomatic each patient is (Dunselman, et al., 2014). So, you could have very few lesions found, but still suffer with significant pain, fatigue, fertility challenges, and other symptoms. You could also have extensive lesions with minimal symptoms. If tissue lesions that are suspected to be endometriosis are found on visualization, they are biopsied, then pathologists determine by histologic confirmation whether they are endometriosis lesions or something else.

Later I'll share more with you of what I tell my patients about how to find the best surgeon for them and some questions to ask yourself to see if surgery is necessary as a part of your healing journey. Surgery is not for everyone, and you always have the option of choosing not to have it. However, for many people with endometriosis a well-executed excision surgery done by an experienced surgeon makes a massive difference to their healing and quality of life. Thus, even if you prefer using primarily natural healing methods, which can be highly effective, don't completely rule out the value of excision surgery yet.

CHAPTER 5

Are *All* of My Symptoms Caused by Endometriosis?

It's very common for people with endometriosis to also struggle with other health challenges. Experiencing symptoms of these comorbidities can give you and your healthcare team more clues about your endometriosis and how to relieve more of your symptoms from the root cause. Thus, while endometriosis may not be causing all of your symptoms, often many of them – even if they seem unrelated – have a similar root cause that can be minimized using the nutrition and lifestyle medicine strategies that you'll learn in this book.

Endometriosis and Digestive Symptoms

Endometriosis can wreak havoc on your digestive system. Because of how endometriosis affects digestive function, these can be the symptoms that show up earliest, which is part of what makes diagnosis confusing as you head down a rabbit hole of seeing gastrointestinal specialists and taking lots of medications for your digestive symptoms. For many girls in pre-puberty with endometriosis this looks like severe stomachaches, including nausea, vomiting, dizziness, and headache. Because inflammation can worsen the impacts of the endometriosis lesions, the stomach pain can be worse with stress or eating some foods. In addition to stomach pain, other common digestive symptoms of endometriosis include heartburn, bloating, slow gastrointestinal motility, constipation, diarrhea, or irritable bowel syndrome.

Endometriosis and Mental Health

Understandably, women with endometriosis who experience high pain levels have a higher incidence of mental health issues (Teng et al., 2016).

Endometriosis is correlated with higher rates of depression. Fifty-nine percent of patients with endometriosis were affected by at least one psychiatric disorder with a significant correlation with their pain symptoms (Vannuccini, et al., 2017). Patients with severe pain showed a higher incidence of multiple psychiatric diagnoses and somatoform disorders than those with mild pain.

One study compared 110 patients with surgically diagnosed endometriosis – seventy-eight with pelvic pain and thirty-two without pelvic pain, with sixty-one healthy controls. All of the subjects completed two psychometric tests assessing quality of life, anxiety, and depression. The worst scores on mental health and quality of life measures were from those women with non-menstrual pelvic pain (Facchin, et al., 2015).

Thus, if you're experiencing depression, anxiety, or other mood related symptoms, know that this is common among people with endometriosis. As you start taking steps to reduce your endometriosis related inflammation, pain, and other symptoms, your mental health symptoms can improve as well.

Endometriosis and Chronic Disease

Endometriosis is also associated with a higher risk of a wide variety of chronic diseases, including:

- diabetes
- pelvic inflammatory disease
- cardiovascular disease
- chronic liver disease
- rheumatic disease
- hypertension and hyperlipidemia
- ovarian and breast cancers
- cutaneous melanoma
- asthma
- some autoimmune cardiovascular and atopic diseases (Teng et al., 2016 & Kvaskoff, et al., 2015)

Interestingly, those with endometriosis are at decreased risk of cervical cancer (Kvaskoff, et al., 2015).

What's useful about knowing the relationship between endometriosis and chronic disease is that as you improve the health of your physiologic systems (like your digestive, immune, and nervous systems) overall, your chronic disease risk can also improve. If you're already struggling with one or more of the above chronic diseases, addressing your endometriosis in a holistic way will often help you reduce, resolve, or recover more easily from your other health issues as well. Even if your chronic disease cannot be completely resolved, you'll be more likely to live with it with a better quality of life.

Endometriosis and PCOS

Polycystic Ovary Syndrome (PCOS) is a state of altered steroid hormone production and activity (Li, et al, 2014). Chronic estrogen exposure and/or lack of progesterone due to ovarian dysfunction can result in endometrial hyperplasia – where the lining of the uterus becomes excessively thick. Several human studies indicate that progesterone receptor-mediated signaling pathways in the nucleus are associated with progesterone resistance in women with PCOS. In endometriosis, at least some of the progesterone receptors are downregulated, also causing endometriotic lesions to become more progesterone-resistant. Thus, for both PCOS and endometriosis, there are likely some common mechanisms of progesterone resistance at the level of the progesterone receptors in the membrane and/or in the nucleus regarding the proliferation of the endometrium. In other words, both PCOS and endometriosis share root-cause challenges in terms of the tissue response to progesterone. In both conditions, there is not an optimal tissue response to progesterone.

For people with PCOS *and* infertility *and/or* pelvic pain, the incidence of suspected endometriotic lesions in controls versus PCOS patients was 12.6% versus 74%, respectively. So, if someone has infertility and/or pelvic pain, and her clinicians suspect that she has endometriosis based on her symptoms, it's far more likely that she actually does have endometriosis *if she has PCOS* (Holoch, et al., 2014).

The results were similar when endometriosis was confirmed by pathology report of the PCOS patients with endometriosis. Fortunately, 76% of the women with endometriosis had earlier stages of endometriosis. However, even more mild looking cases of endometriosis can have significant symptoms and fertility impact. Thus, if you have (or suspect) PCOS and have other symptoms of endometriosis, including pelvic pain and infertility, you have about a 74% chance of having endometriosis compared with those with similar symptoms without PCOS.

Again, like with other chronic diseases, using a holistic approach to healing your endometriosis will also help to resolve your PCOS, or help you to live with PCOS with fewer symptoms and negative effects on your quality of life.

Endometriosis and Cancer

"Endometriosis has the unique status of being a benign metastatic disease. Owing to its ability to invade the surrounding tissues, and in some cases, to metastasize to lymph nodes and beyond the abdominal cavity, endometriosis closely resembles cancer. Despite its destructive and invasive nature, and its clonal origin from single epithelial cells implanting at abnormal locations, endometriosis is not commonly fatal, and endometrial tissue invasion is controlled and eventually stops. However, in some cases, endometriosis can progress to biologically malignant tumors, often in reproductive organs" (Wei, et al., 2011).

Those with endometriosis and their providers need to be aware of the potential progression from endometriosis to cancer. Over 18 years of follow-up, one study identified 228 cases of ovarian cancer in a sample of over 100,000 eligible women, and 166 cases of endometrial cancer among nearly 98,000 eligible women, respectively (Poole, et al., 2017). They found a fairly strong association between ovarian cancer and laparoscopically-confirmed endometriosis. There was a less strong association with self-reported endometriosis. It's possible that many of the patients with "self-reported" endometriosis did not actually have the disease since the only way that endometriosis can be diagnostically confirmed at this time is with skilled laparoscopic surgery. No association has been observed regarding endometrial cancer in patients with endometriosis.

Unfortunately, there is a fairly strong association between endometriosis and ovarian cancer (Wei, et al., 2011). The relative risk of developing ovarian cancer from endometriosis ranges between 1.3 and 1.9 (Somigliana, et al., 2006). The overall frequency of malignant transformation is estimated to be between 0.3% and 0.8%. So, the absolute numbers are small, but endometriosis is a significant risk factor for ovarian cancer, clinically. In populations of primarily infertile women, the relative risk increases to 2.7. The risk of endometriotic-associated carcinoma is higher in older women and in women with genetic predisposition to endometriosis, abnormal inflammatory responses to endometriosis, and long histories of endometriosis.

It's important for those with endometriosis to remain diligent, because ovarian cancer presents with vague symptoms (that somewhat overlap with endometriosis symptoms), it's difficult to diagnose early, and has an overall five-year survival rate of just 45% (Timmons, 2018). The risk of ovarian cancer is another important reason to screen girls earlier for endometriosis, since the longer the history of endometriosis, the higher the risk for ovarian cancer.

What contributes to the increased risk of ovarian cancer in those with endometriosis compared with those who don't tend to progress to cancer? What makes a person with endometriosis more susceptible to cancer (especially ovarian cancer) is a more inflamed physical environment (Wei, et al., 2011). If the environment is less inflamed (potentially because you're eating an anti-inflammatory diet and living an anti-inflammatory lifestyle), the more likely it is that the endometriosis will regress. There will likely still be scarring involved, but at least not a transformation to a dangerous cancerous state.

Endometriosis is also associated with a higher risk of cutaneous melanoma (Kvaskoff, et al., 2014). Thus, people with endometriosis need to be more diligent about using physical blocking sunscreens. I recommend avoiding sunscreens that contain potentially endocrine disrupting chemicals, such as oxybenzone, octinoxate, and homosalate. If you have endometriosis also be sure to optimize your vitamin D levels, and see your dermatologist regularly for skin checks.

Interestingly, endometriosis favors Th2 immune cell production (Wei, et al., 2011). The Th2 immune environment is relatively more anti-inflammatory in some ways, but that's not such a good thing in this case. Ideally, the Th1 and Th2 immune systems need to be in balance. Thus, controlling excessive inflammatory cytokine production (with nutrition and lifestyle) is essential.

But we also don't want the immune system to be too Th2-dominant either. When the Th2 immune system dominates, then the risk increases that the immune system allows for the overgrowth of abnormal cells by not killing them off. Combining the flame of increased inflammatory cytokines with the Th2 dominant immune cells which allow for more unrestricted growth of aberrant cells is a recipe for cancer growth and proliferation.

Later, we'll discuss more about how to reduce the inflammatory environment while optimizing immune function in general, both nutritionally and with healthy lifestyle habits to keep your cancer risk as minimal as possible.

Endometriosis, Allergy, and Autoimmunity

Clearly, endometriosis is an inflammatory disease and it has some autoimmune components. In a retrospective study of 304 patients with endometriosis and 318 without, the results showed that patients with endometriosis have a higher prevalence of allergies and the coexistence of both allergies and autoimmune disease than those without endometriosis (Caserta, et al., 2016). This is correlation, not causation, but it demonstrates that there could be a similar root cause involved in allergies and autoimmune conditions and endometriosis. For example, elevated TSH receptor antibody titers are associated with endometriosis, many women with endometriosis also present with autoimmune thyroid disease and other specific autoimmune diagnoses (Ek, et al., 2018).

Some of the mechanisms involved in cell-mediated immunity that are related to endometriosis include a diminished cell-mediated response that could facilitate a less coordinated immune response. This is a possible mechanism for ectopic (outside of the uterus) implantation of the translocated endometrial-like cells (Eisenberg, et al., 2012), and even potentially for progression to cancer.

We don't know if this is actually what is happening because in the data the T-cell response tends to be inconsistent (Eisenberg, et al., 2012). What about natural killer cells? They may play a role in the clearance of translocated aberrant endometrial cells from the peritoneal cavity of most women. In endometriosis, there is a decrease in local natural killer mediated cytotoxicity in the peripheral and peritoneal fluid to both autologous and heterologous endometrium. So, that diminished immune response could be allowing the aberrant endometrial-like cells to proliferate outside of the uterus in these women with lowered natural killer cell activity.

The combination of suppressed immune function (such as the natural killer cells not cleaning up aberrant endometriotic cells) with increased inflammation is a phenomenon called counterinflammation. Counterinflammation proposes that inflammation contributes to less coordination of the immune system to control tumor and tumor-like growth of aberrant cells (Vasquez, 2017).

There are also several possible mechanisms under study that describe how endometriotic cells evade leukocyte recognition and immune surveillance (Eisenberg, et al., 2012). So, they're staying under the radar, quite literally, from an immune standpoint.

"Inappropriate inflammation is a prerequisite for the development of immunologic autoreactivity" (Eisenberg, et al., 2012). The challenge in endometriosis is that it is not yet clear whether autoantibody formation in endometriosis is simply a natural response to chronic local tissue destruction, or a pathologic response leading to more generalized autoimmune dysfunction.

Thus, using the nutrition and lifestyle medicine strategies you'll learn in this book, you will have many options of tools and strategies to reduce your overall inflammatory load. Reducing inflammation is essential for healing endometriosis and the associated symptoms that are often a part of having one or more of these common comorbidities. As you'll learn in the next section, reducing your inflammatory load is more than just eating lots of vegetables. (Though that helps quite a bit!) Creating an anti-inflammatory lifestyle includes having a support system at work, as well as addressing your body's need for rest and recovery, balancing stress, and more. Continue reading to learn a wide variety of anti-inflammatory lifestyle strategies to heal your endometriosis and any common comorbidities that you're struggling with, holistically.

CHAPTER 6:

How Can I Hang On To My Job Through Treatment?

I f you're like most women with endometriosis, you've been powering through intense pain, crushing fatigue, digestive symptoms, or all of the above for years, even decades by the time you're diagnosed. So you've likely developed some strategies for showing up as much as possible for important work days. My clients have told me some amazing stories of how they showed up for law school classes, long days of patient care, important internships, and even performing stunts, dancing, or singing during live performances. You've likely done this too – took handfuls of anti-inflammatory medications, crashed for a nap during your lunch break in an unoccupied hospital bed or under your desk, had room service deliver bags of ice to your hotel room during a business trip, packed heating pads in your handbag, wore work pants with stretchy bands or abdominal supports underneath, knew where all of the bathrooms were at a busy airport, or something like that. In other words, you're an expert at pushing through to do your very best to show up with as much energy as you can muster for your job. Any employer would be lucky to have you on her team.

But often employers don't see it this way. They don't understand all that you've overcome just to show up and give that speech, performance, or presentation, to write that report, or be with that patient, or that fourth grader who's struggling with reading. Unfortunately, since the vast majority of workplaces do not accommodate chronic illness well, you have to be your own best advocate until workplaces do a better job.

Ultimately, to feel better at work, you'll need to implement a complete, holistic healing plan, including excision surgery if needed and everything you learn in this book. But in the meantime, I want to help you set yourself up for success at work, even while you're in the healing process.

Don't Chase Symptoms, Optimize Systems

The goal of the healing process, as you implement your healing plan, is to lower your overall inflammatory load, balance your hormones, and optimize the functioning of your nervous and digestive systems. While, in the moment, the symptoms can be intense, the goal of this holistic approach is to optimize your physiologic systems so that your overall symptom load can reduce.

Thus, you'll be using nutrition and lifestyle medicine strategies to have less overall pain, better digestion, more energy, more brain focus, more calm and stable moods, better sleep, and more. As you're healing, it's important to practice energy management and to surround yourself with your personal and professional support teams.

It may or may not be possible for you to find a support team at work. But look around and see who could be there for you on your most difficult days. Is there a person that you work with who could help out and assist you with important projects if you really can't be there? Can you talk with your boss about the reality of your endometriosis and how you're on a path of healing, but that it could move faster with her support? Could you hire an intern or assistant to support more of your less-skilled needs?

To work at your highest level as a person with a chronic illness, you have to think of yourself as a 1950s white male executive. Now, this is just an analogy, but stick with me for a moment.

Imagine you're a Mad Men-esque marketing executive. What are your responsibilities? While you might like to drink a cocktail or two, or sleep with a co-worker during the day, your only real responsibility is your work. You have to finish your presentation, convince a potential client to work with your firm, and execute a project. That's it. You don't have to worry too much about what to wear because you'll wear pretty much the same thing every day. You're not responsible for taking care of the grocery shopping, cooking, care of your elderly parent, your children, any housework, etc.

Do you see where I'm going with this? The first step is to get as much help as possible with anything that is not *essential* to your work. Now, if you're in graduate school, or your first very busy years of your early career, you might be working fourteen-hour days, every day, you might be studying on nights and weekends. You might be already giving most of your energy to your job. Even then, I challenge you to dig deep and delegate more.

Perhaps you can delegate *all* housework, cooking, and shopping for the next two years or so as you heal. Perhaps you can hire an intern or work assistant to help you do background research and event planning, or schedule all of your appointments. You're likely doing something in your life that doesn't one hundred percent have to be done by you. If there is anything you can delegate, this is the time to take it off your plate. I know it's not easy. But you're going to need to commit your energy as much as possible to your healing and your work and a few important relationships, such as your spouse, parents, best friend, and/or children. That's it during this intense healing phase. This phase is not forever, but it's generally between six and twenty-four months, and can be a bit longer depending on if and when you have surgery.

Thus, your first healing strategy is to build your Web of Support. You will need a home team, a work team, and a professional team (such as your physician, nutritionist, and physical therapist). Consider who is already on your team. Who you could ask for more help. And who you could hire for more help. Depending on the severity of your symptoms and the demands of your job, this Web will be more or fewer people, and will be required for approximately six to twenty-four months.

Also, be sure that you have redundancy in your Web. It's great to have more than one person to help with shopping or cooking, to give you emotional support, or keep your appointments organized. Spreading the work will make this easier and allow more of the people in your life who want to help you in a specific way to help. For your partner or parent who has watched you struggle for so long, it can feel very good for them to have something specific that they can do to help along your healing journey, since they likely don't have the skills to do your surgery, and they can't just wave a magic wand to lower your inflammation or heal your digestive system. That is the work that you'll have to do by changing how you eat, sleep, move, and manage your stress.

You can download the Web of Support graphic to help you build your Home, Work, and Professional Webs of Support here: https://integrativewomenshealthinstitute.com/endo-book-bonus

Also, look at how you're being of service to others through your work. Whose Webs of Support are you a part of? If you're a writer, it's your readers. If you're an occupational therapist, it's your patients. If you're a performer, it's those who need your art to laugh, cry, or be entertained at the end of their busy day. If you're a teacher, it's your students. If you're a lawyer, it's your clients.

Your work is essential. See that even as you're healing, if you can still write articles, give presentations, care for patients, perform, or teach children, you are using your gifts in an amazing way, and building your successful career is important, not just for you, but for everyone who you serve with your work in the world. Your career success is one of the most important things about having your health. There are many people in the world who will benefit from your career success. Thank you for your commitment to your health. I know it's not easy, but it is of great service.

CHAPTER 7:

The Endo Undiet – Designing Your Personalized Endometriosis Diet

Designing Your Unique Endometriosis Diet

As a nutritionist who specializes in endometriosis, I have seen many "endo diets" (not to mention interstitial cystitis (IC) diets, pain diets, and vulvodynia diets). Unfortunately, my research and my clinical experience with thousands of patients has shown me that there is no one-size-fits-all food plan for people with pelvic pain related to any of these causes. In endometriosis, often women struggle with deep endo-related pelvic pain, musculoskeletal-related pelvic, abdominal, and back pain, vulvodynia, and painful bladder syndromes, such as IC.

Creating your best personal endometriosis nutrition plan involves several factors:

- How you eat
- Your digestive, immune, nervous, musculoskeletal, and endocrine system function
- Foods to avoid

- Foods to increase in your diet
- Supplements to support your systems' functioning (especially your digestive, immune, endocrine, and nervous systems), nutrient optimization, relieving inflammation, and optimizing antioxidant levels
- Living an anti-inflammatory and healing lifestyle

How You Eat Matters (As Much as or More Than What You Eat)

How to Optimize Your Digestive and Immune Function

Why did I combine your digestive and immune systems? Eighty percent of your immune system is in and around your digestive system. The lining of your small intestine, where the vast majority of your nutrients are absorbed, is as important a barrier to keep bacteria, toxins, and other harmful molecules away from your immune system as your skin. By optimizing your digestive health, you'll not only improve your bloating, constipation, diarrhea, or abdominal pain, but you'll also be improving your immune function. As we learned earlier in this book, your immune environment – maintaining an anti-inflammatory environment with healthy and robust immune cell function – is key to healing from endometriosis, reducing the proliferation of endometriosis, and reducing your risk of certain cancers.

Your digestive function is all of the mechanical and biochemical processes by which your digestive system breaks down the foods that you eat, kills off any bacteria or other microbes on your food, absorbs the nutrients contained in your food, and eliminates waste efficiently and healthfully while also reducing inflammation and oxidative stress.

Chew Your Food

Optimizing your digestive function starts with how and how much you chew your food. Most of us eat in a rush and don't chew our food enough. Since we don't generally eat slowly enough, we don't mechanically break down our food enough.

Your stomach has no teeth. Your only opportunity to mechanically break down food, which is essential for absorbing all of the nutrients in it, is to chew thoroughly in the mouth. For the rarer occasions that someone can't chew, using foods that are already at least partially broken down can be helpful. In this case, and in the case that someone is recovering from illness, injury, or surgery, I recommend foods that are easier to digest and absorb with less chewing. Foods that require less chewing are blended foods like smoothies, blended or slow cooked soups, and/or nutrient supplements such as protein powders and liquid or powdered supplements.

It's really important that you chew your food. The research shows that it's ideal to chew each bite of food at least forty times, especially for hard foods like almonds (Cassady, et al., 2009). For most people in my practice that's challenging. So, notice how much you're chewing your food now, and gradually increase. If you tend to chew each bite five times, try to increase it to ten. Then, slowly increase to twenty, thirty, and eventually forty chews per bite, or until the food just dissolves and you can't help but swallow it.

Hypochlorhydria

In the next stage of digestion, the food enters your stomach (after a generally uneventful trip through the esophagus tunnel). The stomach is designed to be a very acidic environment. For many common reasons – including struggling with chronic pain and/or chronic fatigue, being on proton pump inhibiting medications or other common medications for heartburn for prolonged periods of time, or other stressors – the acidity of the stomach can be reduced. Hypochlorhydria is the scientific term for low stomach acid.

High acidity in the stomach is essential for the digestion and absorption of proteins and for the absorption of some nutrients such as vitamin B12.

It can be challenging to maintain enough acidity in the stomach if you have a stressful modern lifestyle and/or have been struggling with chronic illness for a long time (as have most people with endometriosis). Making enough acid to keep the stomach an appropriately acidic environment to kill off bacteria and properly digest and absorb proteins and other nutrients takes a lot of chemical energy, otherwise known as ATP (Arin, et al., 2017). Making enough ATP can be very difficult if you've been sick, in pain, or fatigued for a long time, as is very common for those with endometriosis. Plus, having surgery and trying to live and work during your recovery are all processes that require a lot of energy.

Thus, it's very common for me to see people with endometriosis in my practice who have low stomach acid.

The gold standard medical test for low stomach acidity is the Heidelberg Stomach Acid Test. During this test, you will swallow a small capsule with a radio transmitter in it designed to record the pH of your stomach as you drink a solution of sodium bicarbonate. This is a useful test, but it can be expensive.

As a nutritionist, I test for low stomach acid in my practice using an empirical test called the Betaine Challenge.

The Betaine Challenge

Start with one capsule of Betaine HCL (600mg–750mg) at the beginning of your heaviest protein meal. Some supplements also contain pepsin, which is an enzyme that is activated by stomach acid to allow you to more easily digest protein. You can also use a separate digestive enzyme supplement with a variety of enzymes to support the digestion of protein, fats and carbohydrates.

When you've taken one capsule of the Betaine HCL supplement at the beginning of your heaviest protein meal, notice how you feel. If you notice nothing or that your digestion feels better, continue taking one capsule at the beginning of your heaviest protein meal for the rest of the week. If you notice any symptoms of heartburn, such as burning in your chest, arms, or back, or other signs of indigestion, stop using the Betaine HCL supplement.

If you feel improved digestion, or you don't notice any change in your digestion, then, the next week, increase the dose to two capsules with your heaviest protein meal each day. Continue for another week, then increase the dose to three capsules at the beginning of your heaviest protein meal each day.

If you start to feel symptoms of heartburn or indigestion at any dose reduce the dose back to the previous beneficial dose. For example, reduce the dose down from three to two capsules where you didn't feel any uncomfortable symptoms, just better digestion.

Rarely, it can take high doses of Betaine HCL before digestion begins to improve. However, I highly recommend working with your nutritionist or physician to optimize your dose. Don't try to do this on your own.

There are some risks to adding Betaine HCL to your nutrition plan. This supplemental acid can contribute to ulcers. Do not do this test if you have a history of ulcers or any inflammatory bowel disease.

Foods to Avoid

Unfortunately, food sensitivity testing does not yet give us very reliable data on whether or not to eliminate specific foods for specific people with endometriosis. (There is some data on creating an elimination diet based on the antibody Immunoglobulin G (IgG) food sensitivity testing that can be useful for other conditions, such as migraines (Alpay, et al., 2010).)

Sometimes IgG, ALCAT, or other food sensitivity functional testing can give us more information about which foods may induce sensitivity symptoms for people with endometriosis, if used in context of a good history and clinical assessment. But the gold standard for figuring out which foods are irritating to the digestive and immune systems of any specific person is the elimination diet protocol.

What is an Elimination Diet?

An elimination diet is when you eliminate a group of specific foods that are postulated to include one or more foods that a person is likely to be sensitive to, and thus is likely to be having symptoms related to eating that food. This is not to test for food allergies, which are specific Immunoglobulin E (IgE) antibody-related allergic reactions to food, which could lead to life-threatening anaphylactic shock or other severe symptoms.

It takes three to four weeks to quiet the immune system response to foods that a person is sensitive to, thus it's important that the elimination diet is used as an assessment tool in a committed way for ideally four weeks to get the best information.

This is just a test phase. You will not need to eliminate all of these foods beyond the four week test. Our goal is to make your food plan as varied and flexible as possible. Most of my patients only need to eliminate approximately one to ten foods for the long term, and we can easily adjust the food plan to accommodate for those long-term eliminations.

For now, the focus is on calming the immune system and optimally feeding the gut microbiome, and keeping the nervous system down regulated to reduce or eliminate your symptoms and support healing from surgery. It's ideal to start this food plan three to six months before surgery (if excision surgery is in your treatment plan), and then continue your personalized food plan (which you'll develop after you have re-challenged the eliminated foods) for at least two years after surgery, sometimes longer.

The elimination phase is just four weeks, and then we'll shift to the re-challenge phase.

Your first step is to commit to do a *complete elimination* of a group of foods that have the possibility of exacerbating your symptoms for *four weeks.*

You can do this!

Which Foods to Eliminate for the Four Week Elimination Phase?

For everyone with endometriosis:

- Alcohol
- Caffeine
- Dairy
- Gluten
- Soy
- Sugar/ Sweetener (even natural sweeteners like honey or maple syrup)
- Peanuts
- Corn
- Eggs (Many people with endometriosis can tolerate eggs, but a few can't. So, unless you're a vegetarian and fairly sure that you're not sensitive to eggs, I recommend eliminating them, just for these four weeks.)
- Processed meats (Except for nitrate-free cold cuts.)
- Trans fats or partially hydrogenated oils
- Processed flours
- Fast foods

In addition, some people with endometriosis have difficulty tolerating foods that are high in histamine, so consider eliminating these foods that are high in histamines, histamine-releasing foods, or foods that block the enzyme that breaks down histamine – the DAO enzyme. If you tend to have hives, allergies, or bladder pain, you may have an intolerance to histamine, so try also avoiding these foods during the four-week elimination phase.

- Alcohol
- Fermented foods – sauerkraut, kefir, yogurt, kombucha, etc.
- Cured meats
- Dried fruit
- Soured foods, such as sour cream or sourdough bread
- Aged cheese
- Baker's Yeast
- Nuts
- Avocados
- Eggplant
- Spinach
- Tomatoes
- Smoked fish – sardines, tuna, anchovies, mackerel, and mahi-mahi
- Bananas
- Chocolate
- Papaya
- Pineapple
- Shellfish
- Strawberries
- Preservatives and food dyes
- Black tea
- Green tea
- Energy drinks

Others with endometriosis also have difficulty tolerating foods that can increase autoimmunity. I most commonly see the need to eliminate some of these foods in women with autoimmune disease related symptoms and vulvar or vaginal pain conditions, such as vulvodynia.

- Grains
- Nuts
- Beans and legumes
- Nightshade vegetables (white potatoes, tomatoes, eggplant, bell peppers, tomatillos, pepper spices, cayenne pepper, paprika)
- In addition, avoid the following if you have bladder pain or interstitial cystitis:
- Vinegars
- Citrus fruits and vitamin C supplements
- Foods high in oxalates (spinach, rhubarb, almonds, cashews, potatoes, beets, cocoa powder, okra, raspberries, sweet potatoes)
- Excess salt
- Foods above that are high in histamines

Considerations for Vegans/ Vegetarians

While this elimination phase is easier for those who eat meat, vegans and vegetarians can also do this as long as you include pea/rice protein powder, beans, legumes, rice, and/or quinoa for protein. Including eggs can also be helpful for vegetarians.

Using this type of elimination plan has been shown to work well for vegetarians suffering from vulvodynia (Drummond,

2018), and clinically, it's also useful in endometriosis. The only risk is that you might actually be sensitive to beans, legumes, rice, or quinoa. So, if your symptoms don't improve on the vegan/ vegetarian form of this elimination phase, which will include beans, legumes, rice and quinoa, consider that trying to eat meat and/or fish and testing whether or not you're sensitive to beans, legumes, rice, or quinoa could give you more information about your sensitivities.

Foods to Enjoy!

Here we are, the section you've been waiting for! Here are the foods for you to learn to cook with and eat more of to make your food plan delicious, nourishing, and healing! Enjoy!

Rather than focusing on what to avoid, work with the foods outlined below that will nourish your body with essential vitamins and minerals, as well as anti-inflammatory and anti-oxidant phytonutrients. These foods will work in tandem to reduce inflammation and support vital systems in your body.

Sometimes, using specific foods to support specific conditions can have immediate effects that we can feel – fewer painful symptoms, mental clarity, better sleep, improved mood. Sometimes, results are subtler and you may not feel better right away. And that's OK.

Remember, every human body is different and your journey is unique. Be patient with yourself and your healing and know that every nutrient dense meal you eat is healing your digestive tract, and supporting your immune, endocrine (hormones), and nervous (brain) systems during this time of growth and restoration.

All foods for this elimination challenge phase should be organic if possible, especially animal proteins and those vegetables and fruits in the current Environmental Working Group's "dirty dozen" (https://www.ewg.org/foodnews/dirty-dozen.php).

Also, this is not a restrictive diet in any way! Feel free to eat as much food as you'd like in order to feel full and satisfied.

See the Recipes section for ideas and inspiration.

Vegetables (Carbohydrates)

- Asparagus
- Beets
- Broccoli
- Brussels sprouts
- Cabbage
- Carrots
- Cauliflower
- Celery
- Chives
- Cucumber
- Green beans
- Leafy greens – collard greens, kale, mustard, Swiss chard, spinach, bok choy, lettuce, and most salad greens
- Mushrooms
- Onion
- Pumpkin
- Yams and sweet potatoes (Be careful with these if you're sensitive to oxalates.)
- Radishes
- Rutabaga
- Turnips

- Squash – yellow squash, zucchini, acorn squash, and butternut squash

Fruits (Carbohydrates)

- Apples – Gala, Fuji, Pink Lady
- Applesauce – Homemade with Gala, Fuji, or Pink Lady apples
- Blueberries and blackberries
- Coconut (No additives/preservatives)
- Dates (No additives/preservatives)
- Pears
- Watermelon

Herbs and Spices

- Parsley
- Allspice
- Almond extract
- Anise
- Basil
- Caraway seed
- Coriander
- Dill
- Fennel
- Garlic
- Mace
- Marjoram
- Oregano
- Poppy seeds
- Rosemary

- Vanilla extract
- Sage
- Sea salt
- Thyme
- Tarragon

Healthy Fats

- Avocado (Be careful with avocado if you have an intolerance to histamine.)
- Olives and olive oil
- Coconut oil and coconut butter
- Nuts and nut butters (Avoid during the elimination phase if you have a histamine sensitivity or bladder pain.)

Proteins

- Poultry – Chicken or turkey (Preferably organic and pasture raised with no added sugars or other fillers.)
- Fish (Preferably wild caught. Be careful of some fish if you're histamine sensitive.)
- Beef, veal, or liver (Preferably grass-fed and organic.)
- Protein Powder – hemp, collagen (from grass-fed beef), or hydrolyzed beef

A note on meat, poultry, and endometriosis: While the research supports eating less red meat and chicken for women with endometriosis (Simmen & Kelley, 2018), there are benefits to eating high quality grass-fed, pastured, and organic meats and poultry for some people with endometriosis based on my clinical experience and research from Australia (Jacka, et al., 2017). Various studies published in Australia support eating three to four servings per week of high-quality red meat to optimize mood, which in endometriosis is often related to pain due to changes in neurotransmitters that can be improved with eating, digesting, and absorbing more high-quality animal protein.

Meal Timing

As far as meal timing goes, keeping your blood sugar balanced is an important part of this four-week elimination phase and beyond.

Ideally, eat a savory breakfast or protein smoothie within the first thirty to sixty minutes of waking up in order to start your day with energy and blood sugar balance, usually between 6:00 am and 8:00 am. Then, eat lunch about five to six hours later, between 11:00 am and 2:00 pm. Then, eat dinner five to six hours after lunch, between 5:00 pm and 8:00 pm. Stop eating two hours before bed, and aim to be asleep by 10:00 pm each night.

Here's a sample schedule:

6:00 am: Wake up
6:30 am: Savory breakfast or protein smoothie
12:00 pm: Lunch
6:00 pm: Dinner
9:30 pm: Bedtime routine
10:00 pm: Go to sleep

Planning Your Meals

As you're planning your meals, make sure to get protein, fat, and carbohydrates at every meal.

Your meals will generally look like this:

- Approximately fifty percent of your plate will be vegetables in the form of salads, soups, and/or steamed, sautéed, or roasted vegetables. If you're very fatigued, having a hard time absorbing nutrients, have gastrointestinal symptoms, or are recovering from surgery, most of your vegetables should be cooked and/or blended.

- About twenty-five percent of your plate will be animal (or plant, if vegan or vegetarian) protein. Don't forget to chew thoroughly and take your Betaine HCL supplement when appropriate to help with protein absorption!

- The remaining quarter of your plate will be split visually between fat, such as an olive oil-based salad dressing, avocado, or other healthy fat, and a starchy vegetable such as squash, or half to one cup of rice or quinoa (especially if vegetarian or vegan).

Try not to rely on any one food too much during this elimination phase. Use as much variety as possible. Prepare food in advance and time meals every four to six hours so you won't be caught starving before a meal is done cooking. If you are hungry more often, don't hesitate to add snacks, or eat smaller meals every three to four hours. Your priority is blood sugar balance, so don't let yourself get too hungry, anxious, or "hangry" before eating again. Eat for pleasure, nourishment, and satisfaction. Meals will be more satisfying with adequate fat, plenty of fiber, and lots of flavor using herbs and spices.

Tips for Eating Out

- *Do your research*: When possible, choose a farm to table, vegan, or paleo restaurant. It's helpful to research the menu online before you go. Restaurants that focus on special needs tend to be more sensitive to specific diet requests. Call beforehand and tell them your dietary needs and see what they say. Most restaurants are happy to oblige.

- *Talk to the chef:* If you're not able to research the restaurant before arriving, tell the chef that you're sensitive to dairy, gluten, and many spices. Ask that they cook your meat plainly in olive oil and salt and then order a salad or sautéed or roasted veggies in olive oil as a side. If you're not testing nightshades or certain grains, you could also have options like a plain baked potato topped with sliced avocado or olive oil, or plain quinoa topped with olive oil and/or available vegetables.

- *Pack your bags with flavor:* Bring a small bag of fresh basil, parsley, or dried spices to add flavor. With a small, secure bottle, you can carry around a homemade salad dressing (see Recipes section) or a small amount of quality olive oil.

Supplements to Support Your Digestive Function

In addition to Betaine HCL, most of my patients with endometriosis require additional supplementation, at least temporarily, to support optimal digestive function. Work with your nutritionist or physician to personalize your plan using this section as a guide. I like to think of most supplements as crutches. Most supplements you will be using temporarily, for approximately three to twenty-four months. Digestive support supplements are required while you're healing because it can be challenging for your body to make enough of the nutrients and enzymes that you need for optimal digestion. Enzymatic reactions that help with digestion, conversion, and absorption of nutrients take physical energy (ATP). When you're struggling with chronic pain or fatigue, your energy reserves to perform these enzymatic reactions can be limited. In addition, specific probiotic strains can help to optimize the gut and vulvovaginal microbiome for optimal digestion and immune function.

Stomach Acid

To optimize stomach acid, use the Betaine Challenge as detailed above to determine your best dose of Betaine HCL. Once you determine your dose, you can use Betaine HCL supplement support for any protein heavy meal, at your appropriate dose, as needed.

If you need a little bit of stomach acid support, but Betaine HCL supplementation is too strong or contraindicated for you, you can try to stimulate your own stomach acid secretion using one tablespoon of raw apple cider vinegar in eight tablespoons of filtered water before each meal.

Other support supplements for stomach acid secretion include umeboshi plums or tea made from umeboshi plums, Swedish bitters, and/or gentian root (which is often found in bitters).

Digestive Enzymes

You can test for low pancreatic enzyme levels using stool testing. If pancreatic elastase is less than 400mcg/g, digestive enzyme support can be useful. If pancreatic elastase is less than 200 mcg/g, then digestive enzyme support is generally required and may be required for the longer term or permanently.

Culinary spices can be used to support the stimulation of bile secretion and digestive enzyme secretion. For example, curcumin stimulates lipase (the enzyme that digests fat) activity by 80%, and a single dose of mint led to a 43% increase in lipase activity. The dietary intake of whole spices, including ginger, ajowan, fennel, coriander, garlic, and onion, significantly enhances trypsin (an enzymes that digests some proteins) activity, and ginger increases trypsin activity by 133%. In animal studies, an increase in intestinal lipase activity was observed in animals given single oral doses of mint, garlic, onion, ajowan, ginger, fennel, piperine, fenugreek, and curcumin – between 20 and 461%, depending on the spice!

Bottom line... spice up your food for flavor and digestive support! If that's not enough support to optimize your digestive enzyme secretion, use digestive enzyme supplements, especially if you're fatigued or healing from surgery because, like stomach acid, digestive enzymes require a lot of chemical energy to be created.

In addition to digestive enzyme support to optimize your digestion and absorption of nutrients, post-surgically proteolytic enzymes can be used between meals as an anti-inflammatory to help with your surgical recovery. I recommend the specific brand Wobenzym, which has been found to be comparable to NSAIDS for arthritic joint pain (Bolten, et al., 2015).

Small Intestine Bacterial Overgrowth (SIBO)/ Small Intestine Fungal Overgrowth (SIFO)

Small Intestine Bacterial Overgrowth (SIBO)/Small Intestine Fungal Overgrowth (SIFO) is common in people with endometriosis, as is irritable bowel syndrome, which may be related (Vigano, et al., 2018). Breath testing can support the clinical diagnosis of SIBO/SIFO, which usually presents with bloating, usually after eating, or at the end of the day. Constipation, gas, abdominal pain, and slow digestive motility are other common symptoms of SIBO/ SIFO, but bloating is the telltale sign in my experience.

An important note on SIBO/ SIFO: There are only two ways that bacteria, fungi, and other microbes can overgrow in the small intestine. While it's normal and healthy to have a large population of microbes in the gut, these should be located in the large intestine, not the small intestine. Thus, to have an overgrowth of microbes in the small intestine, they have to enter through either the stomach or backwards through the ileocecal valve (the "door" between the small intestine and large intestine, which should only open one way.) In some cases, surgical disruption of or injury to the intestines could also create an opportunity for microbes to thrive in the small intestine.

Thus, if there are generally only two "doors" for microbes to enter the small intestine, to prevent recurrence, we need to be sure that these are functioning well. To prevent microbes from coming in through the stomach, be sure to address hypochlorhydria. To prevent microbes from coming in through the ileocecal valve, use visceral physical therapy to support the opening and closing of the valve and optimal motility of the intestines.

To eliminate the microbes that have overgrown in the small intestine, there are two options, local antibiotic therapy and herbal antimicrobial therapy.

Rifaximin is local antibiotic therapy, which locally kills off the bacteria, while you also address the hypochlorhydria and/or ileocecal valve and/or motility issues. Talk to your doctor about its usefulness in your case.

As a nutritionist, I commonly use antimicrobial herbs in my practice to eliminate the microbial overgrowth in the small intestine, which have been found to be as effective as rifaximin (Chedid, et al., 2014).

Whether rifaximin or antimicrobial herbs are used, it can take more than one course to address the SIBO/ SIFO, and sometimes alternating a course of antibiotics with herbs over time can be more effective. The key to long-term elimination of SIBO/ SIFO is addressing hypochlorhydria, ileocecal valve motility, and intestinal motility. For some women with endometriosis, the surgery can impact the mechanics of the intestines for the long term, so SIBO/ SIFO will need to be actively managed and can more easily recur.

Digestive Motility and The Ileocecal Valve

I recommend two strategies for optimizing digestive motility, which is key to reducing the risk of SIBO/ SIFO and optimizing the environment for a healthy gut microbiome. The first is visceral mobilization with a skilled pelvic physical therapist, and the second is using a motility activating supplement. In the resources section later in this book, I will share with you how to find a skilled pelvic physical therapist to provide the manual therapy and visceral mobilization to support digestive motility. High quality motility supplements contain ingredients such as artichoke and ginger, or *Perilla frutescens* (Buchwald-Werner, et al., 2014, Giacosa, et al., 2015 & Lazzini, et al., 2016).

The Gut, Endometrial, and Vulvovaginal Microbiome

Given the current state of the research on the impact of the gut, uterine, cervical, and vaginal microbiota on endometriosis (and/or the impact of endometriosis on these microbiota), unfortunately there is not a clear "endometriosis probiotic" supplement that will support everyone with endometriosis. Thus, using probiotics to maintain healthy digestive function and to minimize the risk of chronic vaginal dysbiosis, such as Candida infections or bacterial vaginosis, can be recommended on a case-by-case basis, in collaboration with your nutritionist or physician based on symptoms, stool testing, and/or vaginal cultures. Also consider that an IUD device and string can impact the composition of the bacterial communities between the uterus, cervix, and vagina, which should be distinct because the device itself and the string from the device create a sort of bridge connecting these communities.

Bowel Regularity

Having well-formed bowel movements with a banana-like consistency one to three times per day is ideal. If you have difficulty with constipation or diarrhea, and this nutrition plan addressing your SIBO/SIFO and/or gut microbiome does not resolve your bowel challenges, I strongly recommend seeing a pelvic floor physical therapist.

Re-Challenge Phase

After you have eliminated the appropriate foods for you for four weeks, the next step is to challenge each of the foods that you stopped eating to look for an increase in symptoms.

Some foods from the elimination phase are not ideal for anyone to eat, such as sugar and sweeteners, processed foods, preservatives, food dyes, trans fats, processed flours, and fast foods. Thus, I don't recommend doing a re-challenge of these. As much as possible, eliminate forever processed and fast foods, preservatives, dyes, unhealthy fats, and processed flours. Sugar and sweeteners are socially important to several occasions, but they are unnecessary for optimal health. So, eliminate sugar and sweeteners as much as possible, but use them from time to time during special or social occasions as tolerated and desired.

As you heal, your system may become more resilient and tolerate a bit more sugar and sweeteners, but I recommend waiting at least six to twelve months before using them more than once every few weeks or so. Alcohol and caffeine also tend to be tolerated a bit better after a period of healing and building resilience, thus you should continue to avoid these except for sparing social uses for at least six to twelve months.

How to Re-Challenge Foods

Choose a food to challenge. Eat three to four servings of that food each day for four days. Then, take that food back out of your diet for the remaining three days of the week to assess for any delayed symptoms. If you have symptoms during any of the challenge days, or during any of the three following days during the re-challenge week, discontinue that food and consider it a positive test. You are likely sensitive to that food. Keep that food out of your diet for at least six months before testing again.

For example, you have decided to test goat's dairy products. From Sunday through Wednesday, you eat three to four servings each day of goat's milk, cheese, and/or yogurt. You feel well through those four days, with no changes in your symptoms, and you continue to feel well for the rest of the week, even when you have stopped eating goat's dairy for a few days on Thursday, Friday, and Saturday. This is a negative test, and you can begin to eat goat's dairy normally again. I recommend adding it back in gently and rotating it with other healthy foods. Add a serving or two per week of goat's cheese, milk, and/or yogurt.

On the other hand, let's say you challenge gluten a few weeks later. You eat three servings of bread or whole grain gluten such as barley on Sunday. By Sunday night you feel bloated, your joints ache, and you feel brain foggy. This is a highly positive test. You're likely sensitive to gluten, and should eliminate it.

A note about gluten: Because some people have a severe sensitivity to gluten, called celiac disease, before removing gluten from your food plan, I suggest seeing your doctor to rule out celiac disease. Endometriosis and celiac disease can co-present and may be associated with one another at the root-cause level or may influence each other via inflammatory mechanisms (Stephansson, et al., 2011).

A less obvious positive test could look like this: You add almonds back to your food plan for four days, three servings each day. Tuesday, after three days of eating almonds, you start to feel bloated. You continue to feel bloated on Wednesday, Thursday, and Friday, even when you stop eating the almonds. By Saturday, the bloating has subsided, and does not return the next week, during which you have avoided eating almonds. In this case, you are likely sensitive to almonds, but you may be able to tolerate them in small amounts, less often, and with good attention to chewing and taking your Betaine HCL and digestive enzyme supplements.

Foods to Challenge First

Some of the foods on the elimination list are nourishing and can be anti-inflammatory and healing if your unique body is not sensitive to them. Thus, I recommend re-challenging these first.

While you can choose which order you re-challenge foods, here is a recommended order so that you can resume eating foods that are high in nutrients first.

1. Nightshade vegetables. (Re-challenge these one at a time, if you eliminated them during the four-week elimination phase.)

2. Any other eliminated vegetables, such as those high in oxalates or histamines.

3. Any eliminated fresh fruits, one at a time.

4. Any nuts you eliminated, one at a time.

5. Eggs.

6. Fermented foods, one at a time.

7. Dairy products. (Re-challenge one dairy animal food group at a time, such as goat's milk/cheese/yogurt, then sheep, then buffalo, then cow.)

8. Beans and legumes, one variety at a time.

9. Gluten-free grains, one variety at a time.

10. Chocolate. (Dark chocolate is lowest in sugar and highest in antioxidants, thus it's preferred.)

11. Teas, one variety at a time.

12. Vinegars, one variety at a time.

13. Dried fruits, one variety at a time.

14. Baker's yeast.

15. Soy, if desired. I find many women with endometriosis are sensitive to soy.

16. Gluten, if desired. I find that many women with endometriosis are sensitive to gluten.

Symptoms to Look for to Determine Food Sensitivity

- Joint aches
- Increased period, sexual, or pelvic pain
- Headaches

- Bloating, heartburn, nausea, diarrhea, abdominal pain, or other digestive discomforts
- Anxiety
- Increased fatigue
- Brain fog, forgetfulness, or other mental focus symptoms
- Skin rashes or acne breakouts

After you re-challenge each food for a week, wait until any symptoms subside before re-challenging the next food. Any foods that come up with a negative result, meaning that you don't have any symptoms when you re-challenge them, and you are not sensitive to them, you can simply begin to slowly rotate back into your nutrition plan as desired. Track each re-challenge result in a journal to help you keep track of which foods to resume eating normally. Ultimately, the goal is to expand your food options as much as possible for many reasons, including getting a wider variety of nutrients to support your health, ease of eating socially, and for the taste and pleasure of eating.

For any foods that give you any of the above symptoms when you re-challenge them, consider that you're sensitive to these foods (at least for now until your system becomes more resilient). Leave these foods out of your diet for six to twelve months, and then you can re-challenge them again.

The entire re-challenge process will take a few weeks up to several months, depending on how many foods you needed to eliminate to test related to your unique symptoms. Remember that you will have likely eliminated many foods if, for example, in addition to endometriosis, you also have symptoms of histamine sensitivity and/or oxalate sensitivity, such as bladder pain, hives, or chronic allergies.

I know that this protocol can sound overwhelming, but with good support, it's a very educational process that will give you a lot of power over reducing your overall symptom load, and even reducing symptom flares on important days. Food can be powerfully healing medicine. I encourage you to take the time and get good support to discover which foods are most healing for your body. Having this wisdom and this power over your symptoms will be worth it!

CHAPTER 8:

Fine Tune Your Endometriosis Undiet and Lifestyle with Testing and Supplements

S ometimes it's not enough to use empiric testing and the elimination diet. Using a few functional laboratory tests with the support of a nutritionist or functional medicine physician can make a massive difference in the success of your healing plan.

Optimizing Your Digestion

You already know that Betaine HCL, digestive enzymes, antimicrobial herbs, targeted antibiotics, motility support supplements, and probiotics can support your optimal digestive function. But decisions about which of these you need, and details like which strains of probiotics will best support you can be sped up by using functional testing.

The two tests that I most recommend in my practice for learning more about your digestive function are the GI MAP and urinary organic acids testing.

The GI MAP gives us more information about which bacteria in the colon are out of balance. This information will rule out infections and give us a better idea of which probiotic strains will be most beneficial. Urinary organic acids testing helps us understand how well your body is able to absorb nutrients. This is important to be sure that you're getting enough anti-inflammatory and antioxidant vitamins and minerals, and it helps us see if you have enough resources to build healthy levels of brain neurotransmitters. Urinary organic acids testing also provides us with the best information about whether or not you have yeast overgrowth in your body.

Sometimes other lab tests also add information about nutrient absorption such as your iron, ferritin, and vitamin D levels. The standard complete blood count (or CBC) can add even more information about whether or not you might be anemic.

Are Your Hormones in Balance?

While hormone level optimization in endometriosis can be tricky, given that different endometriosis lesions (sometimes even in the same person) can have different hormone receptors, it's important for overall menstrual and reproductive health to support healthy hormone levels and hormone metabolism.

Endogenous estrogen, for example, is metabolized primarily by the liver, and its metabolites are ideally fully excreted in the urine, and exogenous estrogen is metabolized and excreted via the colon and with your bowel movements. It is common in endometriosis for estrogen metabolism to be sluggish, which can be related to below optimal liver function, dehydration, constipation, and/or gut dysbiosis, which can increase period pain, breast tenderness, and headaches. Thus, looking at lab tests that show the stress that the liver is under, and looking for the genetic single nucleotide polymorphisms (SNPs) that may be making estrogen metabolism more difficult can be helpful. There is not yet a gold standard software to analyze the clinical impact of nutrition related genetic variations, but there are several currently on the market that can be informative. And measuring for your overall environmental toxic load, above and beyond conventional testing (Pizzorno, 2015) can also provide information about unexamined toxin exposures that might be related to your water supply, air quality, cookware, skincare, or other personal care product exposures that can affect your endocrine health. Two of the most commonly used tests are The GPL-TOX Profile by The Great Plains Laboratory and Toxic Effects CORE by Genova Diagnostics.

To get a complete look at your stress hormone, cortisol, and your reproductive hormones, including estrogen, testosterone, and progesterone, and their metabolites, consider the Dried Urine Test for Comprehensive Hormones (DUTCH test) from Precision Analytical. I also recommend that any of my clients with endometriosis have a complete thyroid panel monitored regularly. This panel includes looking at the following bloodwork: thyroid stimulating hormone (TSH), thyroxine (T4), triiodothyronine (T3), reverse T3 (rT3), and thyroid antibodies. Because endometriosis often presents along with other disorders that are autoimmune in nature, and Hashimoto's hypothyroidism is a very common autoimmune disease, this is one to watch carefully. Work with your nutritionist or physician to understand how your hormone levels can be optimized nutritionally based on the results of your hormone testing.

Anti-inflammatory and Antioxidant Nutrients

The most common test that I recommend that my clients use to get a snapshot of their overall inflammation is a high sensitivity C-reactive protein test, otherwise known as the hsCRP. C-reactive protein (CRP) is a protein that is produced by the liver in response to inflammation, thus it is a good measure of a person's overall inflammatory load.

Adding anti-inflammatory and antioxidant nutrient support will aid your recovery from surgery, especially pre- and postoperatively. While there are hundreds of anti-inflammatory and antioxidant nutrients to choose from, those that I use most regularly in my practice, include:

- Fish oil (1000g – 3000g per day)
- L-carnitine (Acetyl-L-carnitine or L-carnitine L-tartrate, 500mg – 2000mg per day, take with fish oil)
- Curcumin (200mg – 400mg per day)
- Magnesium citrate or glycinate (citrate is the most beneficial form if you also suffer with constipation) (150mg – 450mg per day)
- Zinc (25mg – 75mg daily, be sure to also supplement with copper if supplementing with more than 25mg of zinc daily)
- Vitamin D (1000IU – 5000IU per day, take with Vitamin K2)

- L-Glutamine (3000mg – 15g per day for up to three months)
- Demulcent and soothing herbs – such as marshmallow, slippery elm, aloe vera, and chamomile – to support healing of the lining of the small intestine
- Wobenzym proteolytic enzymes (one to two capsules up to three times daily between meals)

Work with your nutritionist or physician to find the optimal combination of supplements and dosing for you.

Estrogen Metabolism Support

While we now understand that endometriosis lesions are not all "fed" by excess estrogen, many women with endometriosis do have excess estrogen, or estrogen dominance (high estrogen relative to low progesterone). To support estrogen metabolism, be sure to address constipation and dehydration first, then consider these supplements:

- If beta glucuronidase is elevated on stool testing (which can cause estrogen to be recycled in the system vs. eliminated), use calcium d glucarate to lower beta glucuronidase levels. (150mg – 250mg per day)
- Diindolylmethane (DIM) (100mg daily, can also be combined with indole-3-carbinol (I3C))
- Broccoli Seed Extract (500mg daily)
- N-acetyl-cysteine (500mg – 1g daily)
- Glutathione (200mg – 500mg daily)

Work with your nutritionist or physician to find the optimal combination of supplements and dosing for you.

Antihistamine Support Supplements

For those who are sensitive to histamine, there are two ways that supplements can reduce sensitivity. One is to add diamine oxidase (DAO), the enzyme that breaks down histamine. The other is to add antihistamine nutrients. Also, be sure to avoid probiotics that produce histamine.

- DAO Enzyme (10,000 HDU – 20,000 HDU daily)
- Quercetin (100mg daily)
- Rutin (200mg – 600mg daily)
- Certain strains of probiotics, including *L. rhamnosus*, *L. saerimneri*, and *L. reuteri* ATCC PTA 6475 (*L. reuteri* 6475), produce histamine and *should be avoided* by those with histamine sensitivity (Liu, et al., 2018)

Work with your nutritionist or physician to find the optimal combination of supplements and dosing for you.

Oxalate Sensitivity Supplements

Remember that some people with endometriosis are sensitive to oxalates, a natural substance commonly found in even healthy foods. To support oxalate breakdown, it's important to have optimal levels of stomach acid (Betaine HCL) and digestive enzymes. In addition, be sure to be optimally hydrated. Plus, add foods high in calcium, reduce sodium, and avoid vitamin C supplements. I recommend getting calcium from food sources because calcium supplementation can increase your risk of atherosclerosis.

Here are some recommended foods that are high in calcium:

- Blackstrap molasses
- Leafy greens (collards, turnip greens, kale, bok choy, mustard greens, etc.)
- Okra
- White beans
- Navy beans
- Black beans
- Chickpeas
- Tahini
- Chia and flax seeds
- Brazil nuts
- Amaranth
- Teff
- Almonds and almond butter
- Broccoli
- Seaweed
- Cabbage
- Brussels sprouts
- Figs
- Black currants
- Blackberries
- Raspberries

As you can see, lab testing and specific supplement support based on your unique needs will make your personal anti-inflammatory nutrition plan even more effective for reducing your endometriosis symptoms. As you use these digestive and immune system healing strategies daily, you will have fewer and less intense symptom flares. Plus, you can increase the dose of certain herbs and nutrients as needed to better show up for days when you must present your best energy for an important event, even if you're dealing with a challenging symptom flare. It's best to work with your doctor or nutrition professional to make decisions about which supplements are best for you. There can be negative side effects for some of these supplements, and there are supplement-drug interactions that need to be considered if you're on any medications.

CHAPTER 9:

Strategies to Help Your Brain Reduce Your Pain

Our brains are powerful pain relievers. There are a wide variety of evidence-based pain relief strategies from pain science education to modulation of neurotransmitters with nutrition to psychosocial strategies like Acceptance and Commitment Therapy (ACT) that involve our brains. There are natural ways to harness these powerful tools without medications. In fact, clinically, I often see that using strong pain-relieving medications as your first tool can make it harder to use these natural brain-based pain relief strategies later.

Sometimes pain medication is literally lifesaving, and it certainly can be quality-of-life saving. If your physician has recommended that you take pain medication and it is working for you, that's great. Plus, it's important not to stop any medications that you're currently using or delay implementing any of your personal health practitioner's recommendations based on this book. It can be dangerous, even life-threatening, to stop some medications without a careful, physician monitored taper. However, I hope that this inspires you to ask more questions and have deep conversations with your physicians and other healthcare providers before you start using pain medications, especially for longer than a few weeks.

For example, in a 2018 review article, *Challenges of the Pharmacological Management of Benzodiazepine Withdrawal, Dependence, and Discontinuation* (Fluyau, et al., 2018), the authors found that "The efficacy of these medications is not robust. While some of these medicines (benzodiazepines) are relatively safe to use, some of them have a narrow therapeutic index, with severe, life-threatening side effects. Randomized studies have been limited. There is a paucity of comparative research." Women with endometriosis have been shown to be more likely to have been prescribed and used opioid therapy long term and in combination with benzodiazepines than those without endometriosis (Lamvu, et al., 2019). The combination of opioids and benzodiazepines is a "potentially hazardous" combination, especially when used outside of the hospital (Hirschritt, et al., 2017).

Gabapentin shows some promise for endometriosis pain management, but it's still only about 30% improvement compared with a placebo (Lewis, et al., 2016). Common side effects include dizziness, drowsiness, fatigue, and a sedated state (which commonly feels like "brain fog" among many of my patients). With increased use of this medication, as the healthcare community works to curb the dangers of opioid abuse and overdose, an increased associated suicide risk is being reported in the literature. A recent study, published in the journal *Clinical Toxicology*, found that intentional suspected suicide attempts associated with gabapentin exposures increased by 80.5% between 2013 and 2017 (Reynolds, et al., 2019).

Other common medications used for endometriosis include combined oral contraceptives and progestins, and other estrogen suppressive therapies (Ferrero, et al., 2018). Each of these options has individual risks, benefits, and side effects. Not all endometriosis symptoms and lesion proliferation are estrogen driven (Brichant, et al., 2018).

Mind-Body Medicine and Pain Science

One of the simplest ways that I explain pain science in my clinic is by teaching the concept of DIMS and SIMS. "DIMS are things that the brain might see as credible evidence of 'Danger In Me.' They may be things we hear, see, touch, taste; things we do; things we think and believe; places we go; people in our life; and things happening in our body" (Butler & Moseley, 2015). In contrast, SIMS are things that the brain sees as signs of safety. Your pain is absolutely *real*. I believe that the symptoms you're experiencing are intense and life altering. And these pain signals are actually coming *from* your brain. We used to think (and learn in our healthcare training programs) that there were "pain receptors" in our tissues and organs.

Thus, if there was damage to a tissue or organ, such as the common example of burning your finger on a flame, you would get a corresponding pain experience. The problem with this theory is that it's not completely true. When you touch something hot that could burn you, there are receptors in your skin that send signals to your brain to move your finger, but that's not the only message that the brain uses to make a pain decision. Ultimately, the decision to send a pain signal comes from a variety of messages that come together in your brain. This is why you could have just been in a very serious car accident, be bleeding, and have many broken bones, and yet experience no immediate pain. In this situation, the pain would just be a distraction from getting you help to try to save your life. In contrast, paper cuts can be extremely painful, and yet there is very little actual tissue damage with having a paper cut.

Endometriosis is the same way. You can have extensive stage-4 disease when your doctor goes in to do surgery, and yet your only symptom might have been mild period pain, or even no pain. But maybe you were struggling with infertility. In contrast, you could have fewer lesions when your doctor goes in to do your surgery, but you can experience severe chronic pain. The severity of your endometriosis does not directly correspond to how much pain you experience.

So, getting back to danger signals (DIMS) and signals of safety (SIMS), you can actively give your brain more signals of safety in order to lower the risk that your brain will propagate a pain signal. Certainly the endometriosis lesions – where they are and their severity – is one part of the equation. Those can be contributing DIMS, and there may be other DIMS that you don't have control over. But let's focus on the SIMS that you can influence.

Signals of Safety to Send to Your Brain to Lower Your Pain Response

Brain health is essential to healing from endometriosis and for reducing or eliminating the endometriosis pain. Pain science is complex. Thus, I refer you to further resources on building an even better understanding of pain science in order to use nervous system based strategies to reduce your pain. The books and resources by Body in Mind (https://bodyinmind.

org/resources/books/), especially *The Explain Pain Handbook: Protectometer* by David Butler and Lorimer Moseley, are great resources for understanding pain science. Dr. Butler and Dr. Moseley explain the need to send the brain "signals of safety" in order to reduce the need for the brain to activate pain signals. From a nutrition and lifestyle perspective, ways to send "signals of safety" to your brain are:

1. *Eliminate dysglycemia (in other words, balance your blood sugar).* Eliminate sugar, sweeteners, alcohol, and caffeine as much as possible. Eat protein, healthy fat, and fiber at each meal and snack. Don't wait too long to eat between meals. Avoid feeling too hungry, anxious, fatigued, or "hangry" before eating your next meal or snack.

2. *Avoid Anemia.* Have your doctor regularly assess your serum iron level, complete blood count, and ferritin level in order to minimize your risk of anemia. The brain needs oxygen to function well, and without good iron stores, the brain will lack oxygen and will be more likely to activate pain signals.

3. *Turn off inflammation.* Inflammation of the nervous system is a "danger signal" that can contribute to your brain being more likely to produce pain signals. Use this anti-inflammatory food and supplement plan to keep inflammation at bay. Have your doctor regularly test your hsCRP level to be sure that your systemic inflammation level is low.

4. *Healthy Neurotransmitter Levels.* In my practice, many women with endometriosis have low neurotransmitter

levels (these can be assessed using questionnaires and urinary organic acids testing.) Specifically, the most common neurotransmitter deficiencies that I see include low GABA, low serotonin, and sometimes low dopamine (catecholamines). These neurotransmitters are involved in pain and anxiety signaling. I find that those with endometriosis, anxiety, and physical pain related to muscular "tightness" most often have low GABA. Those who also have anxiety that involves worried thoughts (more than physical anxiousness) tend to have low serotonin. It is also common to be low in both of these. Those who lack focus, energy, and drive, and/or have depressive symptoms often have low dopamine. Since all neurotransmitters are produced using amino acids (the building blocks of proteins), eating, digesting, and absorbing proteins is essential to having healthy brain neurotransmitter levels. (Refer back to the hypochlorhydria section for keys to protein digestion and absorption.) Until protein intake and absorption is optimized, I recommend specific amino acid supplements as a bridge to calm the nervous system and reduce pain. Learn more about the relationship between amino acids and brain neurotransmitters from my nutritionist colleague, Trudy Scott. (https://www.everywomanover29.com/blog/amino-acids-mood-questionnaire-from-the-antianxiety-food-solution/)

5. *Psychotherapy.*
   - *Acceptance and Commitment Therapy (ACT).* "ACT is a process-based therapy that fosters openness, awareness, and engagement through a wide range of methods, including exposure-based and experiential

methods, metaphors, and values clarification" (Feliu-Soler, A., et al., 2018). If talk therapy is of interest to you, I recommend working with a therapist trained in ACT. You can find a database of trained therapists at: https://contextualscience.org/civicrm/profile?gid=17&reset=1&force=1

- *Trauma informed physical and mental health therapies.* "Post-Traumatic Stress Symptoms have a specific influence on the association between pain intensity and other psychosocial aspects of the pain condition" (Ravn, et al., 2018). Mothers with chronic pain have a higher prevalence of at least one Adverse Childhood Experience (ACE) in their history (Dennis, et al., 2019). Past trauma has a significant impact on current pain. Thus, bringing awareness to and healing trauma through physical and mental health modalities is essential to root-cause pain healing.

6. *Nervous System Calming Practices.* Because pain is so influenced by stress and neuroinflammation I recommend in my practice that everyone with endometriosis find some calming nervous system practices to use *daily*. We live in a fast-paced, stressful modern world. To combat the daily stress and inflammation of modern life, it's important to add daily practices that balance stress and quiet the nervous system. This is even more important during highly stressful times, such as emotionally stressful times, times that you can't eat as well, physically stressful times, during travel, work stress, and/or relationship stress.

- *Meditation.* My personal favorite meditation practice is called Ziva Meditation. I use it myself regularly. Learn more here: http://bit.ly/ZMeditate

- *Prayer.* For many people, simply having a quiet prayerful time each day quiets the nervous system and increases feelings of support and resilience.

- *Social Support.* I recommend that all of my clients complete The Web of Support. (The Web of Support handout is included in our bonuses. See https://integrativewomenshealthinstitute.com/endobook-bonus) Having a variety supportive people in your life – some who laugh with you, some who cry with you, some who eat gluten-free lunches with you, some who take you to the doctor, some who help with your kids, etc. – is essential for nervous system calm.

- *Yoga.* Restorative yoga practices are associated with pain reduction and improvements in quality of life for women with endometriosis (Goncalves, et al., 2017).

- *Sleep.* Sleep is essential for recovery. Get daylight exposure without sunglasses for at least one hour daily. Use blue light blocking glasses at night. Turn off all electronic devices and WiFi in the house by 9:00 pm. Have a bedtime routine, get to sleep by 10:00 pm, and use supplements for sleep support as needed, such as lavender, L-theanine, and melatonin. These are all keys to getting optimal sleep time and sleep quality.

Integrative healing strategies, from brain-based strategies to nutrition, are not always the complete healing solution for endometriosis. In many cases, skilled excision surgery is essential to complete healing and fertility preservation. And generally, having a surgical consult earlier rather than later leads to more successful outcomes.

CHAPTER 10:

Healing My Endometriosis from The Root: Do I Need Surgery?

The gold standard for confirming a diagnosis of endometriosis is laparoscopic inspection with histologic confirmation after biopsy (Kennedy, et al., 2005). Endometriotic lesions are visualized by the use of laparoscope, ideally by a skilled surgeon who specializes in working with patients with endometriosis. It's also important to be aware that the extent of the disease (how many lesions, where they are located, etc.) does not correlate well with how symptomatic each patient is (Dunselman, et al., 2014). So, you could have very few lesions found, but still suffer from significant pain, fatigue, fertility challenges, and other symptoms.

In my practice, I recommend my patients only see expert surgeons who focus the majority of their practice on endometriosis or similar conditions, as I have seen the best clinical results for my patients who get this level of skilled care. See the resources in Chapter 11 for more information about how to find a surgeon who is highly skilled in endometriosis excision surgery.

I also want to share with you what I tell all of my patients who suspect endometriosis and are trying to decide if surgery is right for them. If you have pelvic pain, but are not sure whether or not you have endometriosis, you will need skilled surgery for the proper diagnosis. However, if you will not change how you approach your treatment and healing journey whether or not you have a clear diagnosis, getting that diagnosis may not be necessary. Most of the symptoms of endometriosis can be well controlled in many women with less extensive disease and/or mild to moderate symptoms, without surgery. However, having earlier surgery is essential to reducing the risk of infertility. To decide if having a skilled surgical diagnosis (and treatment) is right for you, consider the following questions:

1. *Is my fertility important to me now or will it be in the future?* If yes, seriously consider having an evaluation with a skilled endometriosis excision surgery as soon as possible to reduce your risk or severity of fertility challenges.

2. *Have I actively participated in skilled pelvic physical therapy, nutrition, mindfulness, and lifestyle medicine with my healing team, but still have symptoms of endometriosis, such as pelvic pain or fatigue that are impacting my life?* If yes, this is another key reason to consult with a skilled excision surgeon. Often, until the underlying disease is surgically addressed, physical therapy, nutrition, and lifestyle medicine will not be as effective for symptom relief.

3. *Have I already had surgery, but it didn't seem to help?* If yes, did you have skilled excision surgery with a surgeon who specializes in endometriosis? Did you have pre-op and post-op pelvic physical therapy, nutrition, mindfulness, lifestyle medicine, etc. to support your best surgical

outcome for at least six to twenty-four months? This level of specialist care is commonly required to get the best possible healing results for endometriosis, especially in complicated cases that may involve bladder pain, gastro-intestinal dysfunction, dyspareunia, fertility challenges, and/or other comorbidities.

Once you have considered these questions, and answered them for your unique circumstances, you're ready to move forward to building your healing team. This will often include consulting with a skilled excision surgeon.

CHAPTER 11:

Relieving Endometriosis is a Team Sport – Who Should be on My Team?

Surgery

When you're on the path of endometriosis diagnosis, treatment, and symptom management, having specific skilled professionals on your team will give you the best possible results.

Because the diagnosis of endometriosis can only be made surgically, since biomarkers and imaging are of limited usefulness at this time, it's essential to consult with an endometriosis excision surgeon to be a part of your clinical team (especially if you answered "yes" to any of the questions about whether or not you should pursue a surgical consult in the previous section). Sometimes ultrasound, MRI, or CT images look fine, but skilled excision surgeons can still find extensive stage-4 disease once surgery is performed.

A skilled endometriosis excision surgeon is the most qualified person to give you a clear diagnosis and perform excision surgery to remove the lesions. Excision surgery is the gold standard treatment for removing endometriosis lesions (Healey et al., 2014). Unfortunately, most gynecologists are not skilled in excision surgery. Working with a surgeon who is specialized in endometriosis will give you the best results.

It's not always necessary to have surgery. But it's always a good idea to consult with an endometriosis expert surgeon to consider the risks and benefits of surgery in your unique case. Every case of endometriosis is unique and individual. Some women have more extensive disease. Some women have more intense or disruptive symptoms. Some women have serious impacts to their fertility. Some women have more cancer risk factors. Every case is different.

In my practice, I always recommend consulting with an endometriosis surgeon sooner rather than later because the earlier you have surgery, the more benefits there are for fertility preservation. Plus, the more quickly you can reduce or relieve your symptoms, the less impact there will be to the nervous system, which increases the potential benefits of pain relief. However, surgery is not always necessary for symptom relief. While surgery can be important for fertility preservation and can significantly improve symptoms, you may be able to manage or even eliminate your symptoms of endometriosis, such as pain and fatigue, by using nutrition therapy and physical therapy alone.

How to find a skilled endometriosis surgeon? The best global directory of skilled endometriosis excision surgeons is the Nancy's Nook Facebook Group. Additionally, I have personally worked with many excellent surgeons in the United States. Connect with a Nook surgeon, or any of the surgeons below for more information:

Nancy's Nook: https://www.facebook.com/groups/NancysNookEndoEd/

Here are other skilled excision surgeons to explore, follow, and connect with for more information:

- http://centerforendo.com/
- http://www.nycrobotic.com/
- https://www.lagyndr.com/
- https://www.womenscentre.net/provider/john-f-dulemba-md-facog
- https://www.mountauburnhospital.org/find-a-provider/profile/malcolm-mackenzie/
- https://www.virginiagyn.com/doctors/dr-kenneth-barron/
- https://www.instagram.com/endometriosis_surgeon/

Pelvic Health Physical Therapy

Pelvic health physical therapy addresses the common myofascial and musculoskeletal pain, plus the post-operative scar management of endometriosis and endometriosis excision surgery.

Below are a variety of directories to help you find a pelvic health physical therapist in your community. Be sure to ask your perspective pelvic health physical therapist if she has post-graduate training and experience with working with those with endometriosis.

- http://endodirectory.com/
- https://pelvicguru.com/directory/
- https://pelvicrehab.com/
- https://ptl.womenshealthapta.org/

Functional Nutrition Professional

Unfortunately, there are few nutrition professionals who are well versed in endometriosis. But our organization trains healthcare professionals around the world to be more skilled in using nutrition and lifestyle medicine to support healing from endometriosis excision surgery and reducing the symptoms of endometriosis. You can find professionals who have done training with our institute, The Integrative Women's Health Institute, here. Remember, be sure to do your own research to be sure that the professional that you choose to work with is the right fit for you.

- http://endodirectory.com/

Pain Management Medicine

There are some pain management physicians who specialize in working with women with pelvic pain. Talk to your surgeon for referrals, or connect with and follow these physicians for more information:

- https://www.instagram.com/pelvicrehabilitation/
- https://www.instagram.com/drtayahmed/

Pelvic Pain Specialist Psychology and Coaching

In addition to The Integrative Women's Health Institute directory above, here are some psychologists and coaches who specialize in working with pelvic pain:

- The IWHI Health Coach Team (the team that I specifically trained to coach clients with endometriosis to use nutrition and lifestyle medicine for relieving symptoms of endometriosis): http://endodirectory.com/
- Alexandra Milspaw: https://4dcounseling.com/our-providers/alexandra-milspaw-phd-m-ed-lpc/
- Lorraine Faehndrich: https://radiantlifedesign.com/

CHAPTER 12:

Endometriosis Can Be Tough on Your Career, But You're Stronger

Endometriosis is a tough disease that is not fully understood, but you have already shown how tough you are. You have a history of powering through your pain. Now, you need to gently shift your mindset to give yourself some space, ask for help, build your Web of Support and your healing team, follow the steps in this book, and invest some time in your health. That might mean that for a few months, or even a couple of years, you need to slow down and downshift your work goals. You may need some financial help and to turn your attention to your own nutrition and self-care to start building up your resilience.

The daily nutrition and self-care practices that you learned in this book when used every day for weeks, months, and years will yield big improvements in your health and symptoms. You may also need medications and/or surgery to keep some of your toughest symptoms under control. And you may need to learn to use specific supplements or other strategies at higher doses or with more support if you have a symptom flare or experience a new stressor.

I know you can do this! People with endometriosis are strong. You have already demonstrated that. You've overcome doctors ignoring you, friends thinking that you were exaggerating your pain, and working through intense fatigue, pain, and anxiety. This program is designed to give your body the nourishment, support, rest, and powerful anti-inflammatory strategies it needs to improve your health from the root cause. You can do this!

Don't expect this to be easy to do on your own. It takes time, a long-term commitment, and gets the best results in collaboration with your personal Web of Support and team of healers. There is a lot of information in this book, and a lot of details that can vary from person to person. You have the steps, but they are not always easy to navigate. Most of us don't have the luxury of healing on a long-term vacation to the beaches of Bali with a personal chef and someone to take care of everything back home. We have to do this in the real world. Most people have to do this while also working at least part time, taking care of children or other family members, continuing to take classes, and all of our other responsibilities. You have the tools here, but the secret sauce to making this work in the real world is getting skilled, caring, and wise support.

Fortunately, you don't have to do this alone. We offer health coaching, specifically for those with endometriosis, to learn to use all of these tools with guided support, coaching, and resources. We'll help you when you're confused about whether or not you should eat nightshades or nuts. We'll help you research the best pain doctors and excision surgeons in your area. We'll help you find a skilled pelvic physical therapist and help you to talk with her if you have questions you're not sure how to ask. We'll give you resources to get the lab testing that you need to fine tune your supplement plan, and hold you accountable to getting yourself the rest and sleep you need, even if you have to navigate a business trip, an important exam or a meeting along the way.

Sometimes fears crop up that this "won't work for me," or "this is too hard." But I have seen this approach work thousands of times. This is not a magic wand. But it is a method specifically designed to address your endometriosis related symptoms and all of the common comorbid symptoms as well. When you focus on root-cause healing, you learn to build your physical and emotional resilience. So, even if you still have symptom flares from time to time, you have more tools, more support, and more clarity about how to navigate those flares. You'll learn the wisdom in your body's messages that will remind you when it's time to rest and when you need to get focused with your nutrition or have stronger boundaries.

Endometriosis is a tough disease, but it's rooted in inflammation and the body's response to having to deal with so much pain and physical stress (on top of the emotional, environmental, and mental stress of modern life). Fortunately, there are powerful anti-inflammatory tools in nature, food, sleep, living your purpose, and working to build healthy relationships. Committing to creating an anti-inflammatory life will not only positively impact your endometriosis symptoms, that commitment will support your ability to do your life's work. Sometimes we think that our role is to work to others' expectations or to push ourselves to work until we can't anymore. But much of your most creative, inspired, and productive moments will actually come from learning to listen to the messages of your body, and take care of your body so that you can hear those messages more easily. Sometimes slowing down is essential along the path of productivity.

Endometriosis can derail your career for a while. But you are strong and you are brave. Taking a step back and investing in your health as soon as you can is a long-term investment in your career. As I mentioned, which was surely no surprise to you, seventy-five percent of women with endometriosis feel that they have not reached their life potential because of this disease (Tu, et al., 2019) Let's change that together. Your work is so needed. And you deserve to feel well.

You've Got This!

Imagine what it's going to feel like when you can wake up on most days without pain, with comfortable digestion, a sense of calm, and energy! Imagine your brain fog is clearing. You're empowered with back up plans, supportive people in your life, and nourishing food in your refrigerator. You know what to eat or take when you have a big day ahead. You know what to do to make it easier to sleep soundly, whether you're at home or on a business trip. You have a plan for days when you have an important class, performance, meeting, or presentation. Sometimes you have a flare, but those days are few and far between.

Imagine knowing what foods and supplements calm your inflammation and make healing from surgery faster. Imagine getting clear on how much nature, darkness, sleep, and exercise you need. And imagine knowing how to easily hold your boundaries and ask for help so that you can take the steps that you need to take care of your health as a normal part of your life.

Imagine having a network of professional and personal support who will help you to thrive at work, even on challenging symptom days. Imagine feeling confident when you say, "Yes!" to a new opportunity, knowing that you're taking care of your energy, reducing your inflammation, feeding your self-healing systems, and that you have tools to use your brain to relieve your pain rather than amplify it.

My wish for you is that the strategies in this book empower you to lead your healing journey and surround yourself with people who support your health and career goals concurrently. I hope that you see the value of having your health so that you can keep doing your work. The world needs your unique brilliance. You deserve to have work that you love and to live your purpose. There are thousands of people around the globe who are using these strategies right now to have less pain, fewer symptoms, and many more productive and joy filled days. Endometriosis is tough, but it doesn't have to rob you of your potential. Join us. Take the first step, and know that there is support available to you to make this journey easier. You don't have to do this alone.

Recipes

BREAKFASTS

Transitioning to more savory breakfasts tends to be challenging for many people, especially Americans! Besides the classic bacon and eggs, many people tend toward sweet cereals, fruity yogurt, pancakes, and waffles. But in order to reduce inflammation and heal, it's important to make a shift in thinking and begin to form new habits at breakfast time.

I've added some sweeter options here (which can also be used as desserts), but in addition to these, I encourage you to start eating for breakfast what you would eat for lunch or dinner.

That means, leftover chicken, steak, burgers, turkey, lamb, or fish, plus any leftover or fresh veggies. Sautéed greens, fresh greens, or a pre-prepared sweet potato or roasted vegetables are all good choices.

A note on smoothies: If you're having a smoothie for breakfast, add a small amount (about a palm-size) of animal protein on the side. Grilled chicken, plain rotisserie chicken, burger, baked fish, nitrate-free sausage, etc.

Creamy Cashew Milk

Makes about 5 cups

Ingredients

1 cup raw cashews, soaked for 4+ hours in filtered water

4 cups water (use less water for creamier milk)

3 medjool dates, pitted

2 teaspoons vanilla extract

Dash of sea salt

Pinch of cinnamon (optional)

Instructions

1. Soak cashews in filtered water for 4 hours or overnight. Drain soaking water and rinse.
2. Add the cashews, water, dates, vanilla, sea salt, and cinnamon to a high-speed blender.
3. Blend slowly at first, then on high until cashews are completely liquefied. This can take up to two minutes.
4. Cashews tend to blend completely, but feel free to strain the liquid through a fine mesh strainer or cheesecloth.
5. Store the milk in a sealed container. It should keep for up to one week.

Berry Breakfast Smoothie

Makes 1 serving

Ingredients

1 serving approved protein powder (see Resources)

1 cup organic blueberries

1 cup spinach or kale, packed

½ avocado

¾ cup almond or cashew milk, or 1 cup water and a small handful of almonds or cashews

1 tablespoon coconut oil

Instructions

1. Combine all ingredients and blend until smooth.

Pear Spice Smoothie

Makes 1 serving

Ingredients

2 tablespoons collagen or vanilla protein powder

1 pear, cored and diced

½ teaspoon ground cinnamon (optional)

¼teaspoon allspice

1 teaspoon vanilla

½ cup cashews

¾ cup water

1 cup ice

1 tablespoon coconut oil

Instructions

1. Combine all ingredients and blend until smooth.

Watermelon Slushy

Makes 1 serving

Ingredients

1 cup seedless watermelon, diced

½ cucumber

½ cup ice

½ apple, cored (optional)

Instructions

1. Combine all ingredients and blend until smooth.

Watermelon Coconut Cream Smoothie

Makes 1 serving

Ingredients

1 serving approved vanilla protein powder (see https://
integrativewomenshealthinstitute.com/endobook-bo-
nus for recommendations)

2 cups seedless watermelon, cut into chunks

½ apple

½ cup full fat coconut milk

½ cup almond milk

2 cups ice (optional)

Instructions

1. Combine all ingredients and blend until smooth.

Vanilla Nut Granola

Makes about 5 servings

Ingredients

½ cup shredded coconut

2 cups almond slivers

1 cup cashew pieces

1 cup cooked quinoa

1 ½ teaspoons cinnamon (optional)

¼ teaspoon allspice

Dash of sea salt

3 tablespoons coconut oil

¼ cup maple syrup

2 teaspoons vanilla

Instructions

1. Preheat oven to 325°F.
2. Mix all ingredients together in a large bowl.
3. Spread evenly onto a large baking sheet.
4. Bake for 20 minutes on 325°F, stirring occasionally. Make sure it doesn't burn!
5. Raise temperature to 350°F, stirring occasionally. Make sure it doesn't burn!
6. Stir granola and bake for another 10 minutes at 350°F.
7. Eat with coconut yogurt (recipe below) and homemade berry compote (recipe in Desserts section), or simply enjoy with unsweetened coconut yogurt, almond milk, hemp milk, or cashew milk.

Coconut Yogurt

*You can also purchase dairy-free, unsweetened yogurt from the store.

Makes 1 quart

Ingredients

2 (14 ounce) cans full fat coconut milk

4 teaspoons grass-fed gelatin

4 probiotic capsules

2 tablespoons maple syrup (optional)

Equipment

Glass jars with lids, for storing the yogurt

Measuring spoons

Medium saucepan

Whisk

Thermometer

Instructions

1. Warm the oven until it reaches about 100°F. Turn off the heat and leave the oven light on to help keep the oven warm.
2. Sterilize jars by washing in the dishwasher or rinsing them with boiling water.
3. Pour the coconut milk into a medium saucepan over low and stir until smooth. Do not bring to a boil.
4. Scoop a quarter cup of the warm coconut milk into a bowl and stir in the gelatin until it's fully dissolved, then pour back into the pot.
5. Warm the coconut milk until it starts to simmer. Whisk and turn heat down to low. Continue on low for 5–10 minutes, whisking continuously.
6. Cool the milk mixture until it's 100°F or just warm to the touch.
7. Open the probiotic tablets and mix the contents into the milk.
8. Add the maple syrup, if using, and stir.
9. Pour mixture into the pre-sterilized jars and screw on the lids. Place into the warmed oven and leave for 12–24 hours.

10. Chill the yogurt in the fridge for a couple of hours – it will thicken as it chills. If there is separation, stir to recombine. Store yogurt in the fridge for up to two weeks.

MAIN DISHES

Eating for healing means that your focus should be on enjoying delicious and nourishing food. No need to restrict calories. If you're hungry, eat. These delicious recipes should make eating to heal enjoyable, flavorful, and relaxing. The following is a testimonial from Termeca Mitchell, 37 years old from Tampa Bay, Florida who tried these recipes after Naja Chikazunga-Martin, PT, DPT, WHC, PRPC, our graduate, recommended this recipe guide to her.

"I'm a mother of three who has been struggling with pelvic pain for years. After having numerous surgeries, I finally thought I was fixed. But in 2017 I began having pelvic pain again, so I scheduled an appointment to see my doctor. He stated that I was fine, so I went about my day. As time passed, the pain started to get worse, so I scheduled another appointment with my doctor, but he wasn't in. I was told I had to see another doctor, who told me that it was normal to have pains in my pelvic area, because even though I had a partial hysterectomy, my body still had the symptoms of a menstrual cycle and that I still ovulate. After that appointment, I thought, 'Maybe that's true,' and just brushed it off. Long story short, the pain began to be unbearable, to the point where it interfered with work and my daily activities.

"My husband and I decided to schedule an appointment with my doctor who performed the surgery. After seeing him, I was scheduled to do pelvic therapy with Naja. When I met with her, she talked with me and sent me an email with a nourishment guide I should try. Due to scheduling conflicts, I missed a couple of appointments but thought, 'Hey, let me try this diet thing.' So I started on the diet Naja sent. During the first week or so into the process, I started to feel so much better, and in six weeks, my pain had decreased. I am now able to perform house chores and have intercourse without pain. I saw Naja for my second visit and was excited to share with her that I had begun an exercise routine of two to three times per week and was enjoying intercourse with no pain." She has since "graduated" from pelvic physical therapy after achieving 100% of her goals in just three visits in nine weeks. She even found a new job. She has continued her new exercise routine three to four times per week, and she can't say enough about how the health coaching and physical therapy experience with Naja, and this nutrition plan changed her life.

Beef and Broccoli with Sweet Potato Noodles

Makes 2 servings

Ingredients

Marinade

 12-16 ounces lean stir-fry beef slices

 2 tablespoons coconut aminos

 2 cloves garlic, crushed and minced

 2 teaspoons fresh ginger, grated

1 teaspoon dried turmeric

½ teaspoon sea salt

½ teaspoon pepper (as tolerated)

Noodles

1 large sweet potato, spiralized

1 tablespoon coconut oil or olive oil (plus, additional oil if needed to cook the broccoli)

Salt and pepper to taste

Sauce

¼ cup coconut aminos

2 tablespoons cashew or almond butter, or ½ cup raw nuts

½ green apple, cored

1 teaspoon fresh ginger, grated

1 clove garlic, minced

Vegetables

1 small head broccoli, chopped

Instructions

1. Preheat oven to 375°F.

2. Place meat and marinade ingredients in a large glass bowl and cover for 30–60 minutes.

3. Meanwhile, make the sweet potato noodles and toss with olive oil, salt and pepper to coat evenly. Bake "zoodles" for 15–20 minutes or until tender. Set aside.

4. In a large skillet over medium heat, add the broccoli and about ½ cup water. Cover and steam for 2–3 minutes, then drain the water and set the broccoli aside.

5. Whisk together the sauce ingredients in a small bowl or blend in a high-speed blender until smooth.

6. Heat 1–2 tablespoons coconut oil in a large skillet or wok. Add meat and brown for 5–10 minutes.
7. Add more cooking oil if needed. Add the broccoli and the sauce and cook an additional minute.
8. Remove from the heat and toss with sweet potato noodles and serve.

Chicken Zucchini Poppers

Makes 2–4 servings

Ingredients

1 pound ground organic chicken breast

2 cups grated zucchini

3–4 tablespoons basil, minced

1 clove garlic

1 teaspoon salt

½ teaspoon pepper (if tolerated)

½ teaspoon coriander

Olive oil or coconut oil for cooking

Instructions

1. Preheat oven to 400°F.
2. Mix chicken, zucchini, basil, garlic, salt, pepper, and coriander.
3. Grease a baking sheet with olive oil or coconut oil and use a small spoon to shape meatballs about 1–2 inches in diameter and place about 1 inch apart. Drizzle some more olive oil over the meatballs.
4. Bake for 20–30 minutes or until cooked through. You can broil for an additional 2–3 minutes to brown.

Grilled Chicken

Makes 4 servings

Ingredients

1 full pastured chicken, cut into pieces, or 2 thighs, 2 breasts, and 2 legs

1 teaspoon salt

¼ teaspoon pepper (if tolerated)

1 teaspoon dried basil

1 teaspoon dried oregano

1 teaspoon dried rosemary

Instructions

1. Preheat your grill to medium-high. If you are using a charcoal grill, coals are ready when you can hold your hand 5 inches above grill for just 3 to 4 seconds.
2. Combine salt, pepper, and all the herbs and rub the chicken with the mixture. (You may not use the entire mixture.)
3. Let the chicken stand at room temperature for 30 minutes.
4. Place chicken on the grill, skin-side down.
5. Close the cover, grill 8 minutes and flip. Grill until chicken is cooked through, about 15 minutes more.
6. Transfer to a plate and let the meat rest for about 10–15 minutes, then enjoy.

Herbed Steak

Makes 1 serving

Ingredients

1 cup packed fresh basil leaves

2 tablespoons packed fresh oregano leaves

1 tablespoon packed fresh rosemary leaves

1 tablespoon packed fresh thyme leaves

1 tablespoon packed fresh tarragon leaves

2 cloves garlic, minced

¾ cup extra virgin olive oil

Sea salt to taste

1 (2–3-inch thick) grass-fed rib eye, strip, or porter-house steak

Instructions

1. Preheat oven to 500°F.

2. Finely chop all herbs and transfer to a small bowl.

3. Mix herbs and olive oil together and add salt and pepper to taste. Set aside for flavors to meld.

4. Rub steak with about 2 tablespoons of olive oil and season steak liberally with salt and pepper if you can handle it.

5. Sear the steak in a hot dry pan for 30 seconds on each side.

6. Then place the steak in the preheated oven for 2 minutes. Flip and cook for another 2 minutes. If you prefer a medium-cooked steak, leave in for 1 minute longer on each side.

7. Remove from the oven and let sit for 5 minutes.

8. Slice steak against the grain and drizzle herb sauce over the top and serve.

Simple Salmon Cakes

Makes 4 cakes

Ingredients

1 can wild-caught salmon

½ cup cooked, mashed sweet potato

Dash of salt

Dash of pepper (if tolerated)

1 teaspoon garlic powder, or 1 garlic clove smashed and minced

½ cup almond flour or almond meal

2–3 tablespoon coconut or olive oil for cooking

Instructions

1. Mix salmon with cooked sweet potato and spices in a small bowl.
2. Add almond flour or almond meal to a separate bowl or plate.
3. Take a small handful of the salmon mixture and form into a loose ball.
4. Roll salmon into the almond flour or almond meal until fully covered and place into the heated oil.
5. Cook for 3–4 minutes on each side or until golden brown and heated through.
6. Place on a paper towel to rest.
7. Add to salads as your protein or eat with roasted or steamed veggies.

Fish en Papillote

Makes 1 serving

Ingredients

1 zucchini, sliced thin

1 shallot, sliced

2 cloves of garlic, smashed and minced

½ pound piece of salmon

1–2 tablespoon fresh dill

Salt and pepper to taste (optional)

Extra virgin olive oil

Instructions

1. Heat oven to 350°F.
2. Fold a 24-inch sheet of parchment paper in half, and cut out a heart shape about 3 inches larger than the fish fillet.
3. Place fillet near the fold, and place zucchini, garlic, shallot, dill, salt and pepper onto the parchment paper. Drizzle with 1–2 teaspoons olive oil.
4. Brush edges of parchment paper with olive oil, fold paper to enclose fish, making small overlapping folds to seal the edges, starting at the curve of the heart. Be sure each fold overlaps the one before it so that there are no gaps. Brush the outside of the package with olive oil.
5. Put packages on a baking sheet and bake for 15–25 minutes, depending on the thickness and size of your salmon. If you have a thinner piece salmon, bake for less time, and if you have a thicker piece of salmon, aim for 25 minutes. Tear open the parchment paper at the table, enjoy the aromas, and dig in!

Basil Burgers with Baked Asparagus

Makes 2–4 servings

Ingredients

1 teaspoon dried basil

1 teaspoon dried oregano

1 clove garlic, minced

1 teaspoon powdered garlic

1 pound ground beef, bison, turkey, or lamb

3 tablespoons coconut or olive oil, divided

7-8 asparagus spears

Instructions

For burgers:

1. Mix spices and ground meat in bowl and roll into 3–4 large balls and flatten to desired thickness.
2. Heat 1 tablespoon oil in a pan or griddle over high heat until the oil begins to shimmer.
3. Cook the burgers until golden brown and slightly charred on the first side, about 3 minutes on each side for beef and 5 minutes on each side for turkey.
4. Serve with all your favorite burger fixings, wrapped in lettuce.

For asparagus:

1. Trim tough ends off asparagus and wash.
2. Preheat an oven to 425°F.
3. Place the asparagus into a mixing bowl, and drizzle with 2 tablespoons oil. Toss to coat the spears, then sprinkle with garlic powder, salt, and pepper.
4. Bake in the preheated oven until just tender, 12–15 minutes depending on thickness.

Unstuffed Zucchini

Makes 2–4 servings

Ingredients

2 tablespoons extra virgin olive oil

2 garlic cloves, minced

1 teaspoon dried basil

1 teaspoon dried oregano

1 teaspoon dried thyme

½ teaspoon sea salt

4–5 portabella mushrooms, sliced

1 large zucchini, sliced in ½-inch thick slices

1 pound ground beef or turkey – less than 10% fat

2 cups cooked rice, pasta, or quinoa

Instructions

1. In a large pan heat oil on medium heat and add the garlic. Cook garlic until just browned.
2. Add the meat and cook through.
3. Add spices, mushrooms, and zucchini slices.
4. Sauté until zucchini slices are fork tender.
5. Serve over the rice, noodles, or quinoa.

Easy Roast Beef with Sweet Potatoes

Makes up to 4 servings

Ingredients

1 (2–3pound) grass-fed beef pot roast

1–2 cloves garlic, minced

1 teaspoon oregano

Filtered water

4 medium sweet potatoes, cut into chunks

4 large carrots, sliced

3 stalks celery, cut in chunks

Instructions

1. Place your pot roast into a heated crockpot with minced garlic and oregano.

2. Add enough water to cover the meat and cook for 4 hours on high.

3. Add the sweet potatoes, carrots, and celery.

4. Continue cooking until veggies are tender and meat falls apart, about 2 hours more.

5. Serve over 1 cup of rice or cauliflower rice with plenty of juice from the roast!

Shrimp and Bacon with Spaghetti Squash

Makes 4 servings

Ingredients

2–3 cloves garlic, smashed and minced

1 pound shrimp

4 strips of bacon, chopped (optional)

4 cups spinach or kale, chopped

Sea salt and ground ginger to taste

1 large spaghetti squash, cooked. (You can also use 4 cups rice, 1 package rice pasta, or 1 pound "zoodled" zucchini).

Instructions

1. Cook the bacon, if using, in a skillet over medium heat until crispy, then remove from the pan and set aside.
2. Cook the garlic in the bacon grease for 3–4 minutes, stirring occasionally. Add the shrimp, greens, squash, sea salt, and ginger and cook until the shrimp is pink, about 5 minutes.
3. Add the chopped bacon and spaghetti squash noodles to the pan and heat through.

SALADS

If you struggle with bladder pain, salad dressing can be tricky since citrus fruits and vinegars can trigger bladder pain flares. Fortunately, all of these salad dressings are bladder friendly. Feel free to bring a small jar with you to restaurants to add flavor to plain salads.

Blueberry Basil Dressing

Ingredients
¼ cup fresh or frozen blueberries
½ cup olive oil or avocado oil
¼ cup packed fresh basil

Instructions
1. Combine all ingredients and blend until smooth.

Sesame Ginger Dressing

Ingredients

¼ cup sesame or olive oil

3 tablespoons sesame seeds

⅓ cup almond butter

½ teaspoon sea salt, or to taste

⅓ cup coconut aminos

1 teaspoon powdered ginger or 1 tablespoon fresh ginger, grated

1–2 cloves garlic, minced

⅓ cup water

Instructions

1. Lightly toast sesame seeds.
2. Combine all ingredients into a high-speed blender.
3. Use the water to dilute the mixture (it will be pretty thick) to a desired consistency.

Honey Pear Dressing

Ingredients

⅓ cup olive oil

1 pear, seeded

½ - 1 tsp honey, or to taste

1 teaspoon vanilla

Instructions

1. Combine all ingredients and blend until smooth.

Italian Dressing

Ingredients

¼ cup fresh basil

1 tablespoon fresh oregano, chopped

1 tablespoon fresh rosemary, chopped

1 tablespoon fresh thyme

2 cloves garlic

¼ teaspoon sea salt

¾ cup extra virgin olive oil

Instructions

1. Combine all ingredients and blend until smooth.

Pesto Dressing

Ingredients

4 cups fresh basil leaves (about 2 large bunches)

¾ cup extra virgin olive oil

3–5 cloves garlic

⅓ cup cashews

1 teaspoon sea salt

Instructions

1. Combine all ingredients and blend until smooth.

Watermelon Salad

Makes 2–3 servings

Ingredients

4 watermelon radishes

1 large cucumber

2 cups seedless watermelon

1½ cups micro greens

Olive oil for drizzling

Sea salt to taste

Instructions

1. Slice radish and cucumber into thin slices.
2. Chop watermelon into uniform cubes.
3. Combine radish, watermelon, and cucumber in a large bowl and add micro greens.
4. Drizzle with olive oil and sea salt to taste.

Quinoa Salad

Makes 4 servings

Ingredients

2 cups quinoa, uncooked

1 medium pear, cut into bite-sized chunks

1 cup carrot, shredded

1 cup celery, chopped

½ cup shredded coconut

¾ cup slivered almonds

2 tablespoons olive oil

Sea salt to taste (optional)

Instructions

1. In a medium saucepan, cook quinoa according to package instructions.
2. In a large bowl, combine quinoa with the remaining ingredients and serve immediately.
3. Store in the refrigerator in an airtight container for up to 5 days. Can be served warmed or cold.

Beet Cucumber Salad

Makes 4 servings

Ingredients

4 roasted beets, sliced

¼ cup almonds, sliced

1 cup arugula

2 cups spinach leaves

½ cup cucumber slices

3 tablespoons extra virgin olive oil

Instructions

1. Wash lettuces and dry off. Place into large salad bowl.
2. Slice beets and cucumbers, place on top of salad.
3. Add almond slices.
4. Drizzle oil onto salad or serve by the bowl.

Nori Salad Wraps

Makes 1–2 servings

Ingredients

1 (5 ounce) can low-mercury tuna or salmon

1 tablespoon extra-virgin olive oil

1 tablespoon canned coconut milk

½ teaspoon coriander

¼ teaspoon salt

4–6 nori seaweed sheets

2 carrots, thinly sliced

1 cucumber, thinly sliced

1 avocado, sliced

Instructions

1. In a medium bowl stir together tuna, olive oil, coconut milk, coriander, and salt.
2. Prep veggies and lay out nori wraps.
3. Spoon mixture over nori sheets, top with veggies and roll into cone- shaped wraps.

SIDES

Roasted Sweet Potatoes

Makes 2–4 servings

Ingredients

2 large sweet potatoes, cut evenly into wedges

2 ½ tablespoons olive oil or coconut oil

1 ½ teaspoons salt

1 teaspoon garlic powder

¼ teaspoon dried oregano or 1 teaspoon fresh oregano

½ teaspoon black pepper (optional)

Instructions

1. Preheat oven to 450°F. Line a large baking sheet with aluminum foil and place a baking rack on top. Set aside.

2. Cut off the pointy ends of the potatoes. Slice the sweet potatoes in half lengthwise, then cut each piece into 1 1/2-inch wedges.

3. In a large bowl, mix wedges with oil, garlic, oregano, salt, and pepper. Coat potatoes thoroughly.

4. Arrange the potatoes in a single layer on the baking rack and bake for 30 minutes.

5. After 30 minutes, turn on the broiler and cook for another 3–5 minutes or until brown and crispy.

6. Cool wedges and serve.

Perfectly Cooked Broccoli Rabe

Makes 2–4 servings

Ingredients

Sea salt

1 bunch broccoli rabe, tough, non-leafy stems removed

Garlic-infused olive oil

Cracked pepper (if tolerated)

Instructions

1. Bring a large pot of well-salted water to a boil.

2. Set up a bowl of well-salted ice water.

3. Drop the broccoli rabe into the boiling water and cook for 1 minute.

4. Remove from the boiling water and plunge immediately into the ice water.

5. Once cool remove from the ice water and let dry. It can be used right away or held for future use. (Use in salads, sautéed as a side, or as a snack.)

6. Coat the bottom of a large sauté pan with olive oil and bring to medium heat.

7. Add the broccoli rabe and toss in the oil to heat up. Remember the broccoli is already cooked. Add more oil, if needed, and season with salt if needed (it probably will).

Cauliflower Rice

*You can now buy cauliflower rice pre-"riced" at many natural or whole foods stores. Look in the frozen section as well!

Makes 4 servings

Ingredients

1 head of cauliflower, cut into florets

1 tablespoon coconut oil, olive oil, or bacon grease

Fresh herbs of your choice

Salt and pepper to taste

Instructions

1. Add the cauliflower florets to a food processor and process until finely chopped into "rice" sized pieces.

2. You can store like this in the fridge or freezer or cook immediately.

3. To cook, heat your oil in a large skillet and add the riced cauliflower. Stir constantly, sort of like a stir-fry, for 5–10 minutes or until tender, but it still has a bit of crunch.

4. Add salt and pepper to taste and serve!

Chopped Broccoli Slaw

Makes 4 servings

Ingredients

2 heads broccoli, chopped into small florets (I use the stalk as well)

6 pieces bacon, cooked and chopped into small pieces (optional)

½ cup slivered almonds, toasted

1 cup celery, chopped

1 cup crispy apple (like Fuji), chopped small

½ cup Honey Pear Dressing (see above recipe)

Instructions

1. Prepare Honey Pear Dressing.

2. Prepare bacon by cooking in the oven at 350°F for 20 minutes or until crispy. Let cool, chop, and set aside.

3. Lightly steam broccoli until bright green, about 1 minute. Let cool. (You can also use it raw.)

4. Toast almonds in a dry pan on the stovetop until fragrant and brown, or place almonds on a baking sheet and bake at 350°F for 3–5 minutes, stirring every 30 seconds or so.

5. Combine broccoli, bacon, almonds, celery, and apples in a large bowl. Drizzle dressing onto the salad. Use more or less dressing according to your tastes.

Cabbage Apple Slaw

Makes 4 servings

Ingredients

    5 cups cabbage, thinly sliced

    2 cups Fuji apples, chopped

    2 cups carrots, shaved

    ½ cup olive or avocado oil

    2 tablespoons maple syrup

    Salt and pepper to taste

Ingredients

1. Combine cabbage, apples, and carrots into a large bowl.
2. Combine remaining ingredients in small bowl; stir or whisk well.
3. Add dressing mixture to the vegetables and coat well.
4. Cover and chill for at least an hour or eat immediately.

Roasted Vegetables

Makes 4 servings

Ingredients

    1 tablespoon cooking fat such as olive oil or coconut oil

    ½ pound carrots, chopped

    ½ pound sweet potato, chopped

    1 pound squash, chopped

    ¼ teaspoon ground ginger

    1 teaspoon powdered garlic or 2–3 garlic cloves, smashed and minced

    ¼ teaspoon sea salt

    Cracked pepper to taste (as tolerated)

Instructions

1. Preheat the oven to 400°F.
2. Toss the vegetables with the cooking fat, salt, pepper, and spices.
3. Place in large baking dish. Cover the dish with foil and then bake for 15–20 minutes until the vegetables are mostly cooked.
4. Uncover, stir, and cook until the vegetables are fork tender.

DESSERTS

Eating to heal includes dessert! While too much sugar can be inflammatory and contribute to pain, lightly sweetened desserts with a focus on anti-inflammatory fruits and healthy fats are a delicious way to nourish your brain and hormone and immune systems.

Layered Fruit Parfait

Makes 2 servings

Ingredients

    2 cups Coconut Yogurt (see recipe)
    1 cup Granola (see recipe)
    Blueberry Compote (see recipe below)

Blueberry Compote
Ingredients

    1 tablespoon grass-fed butter or coconut oil
    2 cups blueberries

2 teaspoons vanilla

1 tablespoon maple syrup

Instructions for compote:

1. Melt butter into a small saucepan.
2. Add berries, vanilla, and maple syrup.
3. Warm on medium heat, stirring constantly for about 10 minutes or until mixture has combined.

Instructions for parfait:

1. Layer the yogurt, granola, and compote in a small glass, repeating 2–3 times and enjoy!

Nutty Apple Pie Crumble

Makes 4–6 servings

Ingredients

6 medium size apples, diced

2 cups almond flour

½ cup coconut oil

¼ cup maple syrup

1 ½ teaspoons vanilla extract

1 teaspoon ground cinnamon (optional)

½ teaspoon allspice

Instructions

1. Preheat oven to 350°F and lightly grease a pie pan with coconut oil.
2. Whisk together the maple syrup, vanilla extract, cinnamon, and allspice in a bowl. Add the flour and whisk until smooth and combined.

3. Cut in the coconut oil and stir with a fork until it forms a crumbled mixture.

4. Spread the apples in the bottom of the pie pan and top with the crumbled mixture.

5. Cover with foil then bake for about 45 minutes until the apples are tender. Remove the foil and bake for another 10 minutes. Let cool for 10 minutes before serving.

SNACK IDEAS

Apple slices and almond butter

Pear slices and cashew butter

Celery and chopped carrots dipped in blended avocado

Sliced roast turkey with an apple

Paleo granola (see recipe above in the Breakfast section)

Olives and sliced roast beef

Coconut milk ice cream topped with sliced almonds, or blueberries.

Coconut yogurt parfait (see recipe above in the Dessert section)

Nori Salad Wraps (see recipe above in the Salad section)

References

Adamson, G.D., et al. (2010). Creating solutions in endometriosis: global collaboration through the World Endometriosis Research Foundation. *J of Endometriosis*, 2(1):3-6.

Alghetaa, H.F., Mohammed, A., Nagarkatti, M., & Nagarkatti. (2018). Gut dysbiosis and immunological profile in endometriosis. *J Immunol*, 200 (1 Supplement) 108.6.

Alimi, Y., Iwanaga, J., Loukas, M., & Tubbs, R. S. (2018). The Clinical Anatomy of Endometriosis: A Review. *Cureus*, 10(9), e3361. doi:10.7759/cureus.3361

Alpay, K., Ertas, M., Orhan, E. K., Ustay, D. K., Lieners, C., & Baykan, B. (2010). Diet restriction in migraine, based on IgG against foods: a clinical double-blind, randomised, cross-over trial. *Cephalalgia: an international journal of headache*, 30(7), 829–837. doi:10.1177/0333102410361404

Anderson, G. (2019). Endometriosis Pathoetiology and Pathophysiology: Roles of Vitamin A, Estrogen, Immunity, Adipocytes, Gut Microbiome and Melatonergic Pathway on Mitochondria Regulation. *BioMol Concepts*, 10, 133–149. https://doi.org/10.1515/bmc-2019-0017

Arin, R. M., Gorostidi, A., Navarro-Imaz, H., Rueda, Y., Fresnedo, O., & Ochoa, B. (2017). Adenosine: Direct and Indirect Actions on Gastric Acid Secretion. *Frontiers in physiology*, *8*, 737. doi:10.3389/fphys.2017.00737

Ata, B., Yildiz, S., Turkgeldi, E., Brocal, V. P., Dinleyici, E. C., Moya, A., & Urman, B. (2019). The Endobiota Study: Comparison of Vaginal, Cervical and Gut Microbiota Between Women with Stage 3/4 Endometriosis and Healthy Controls. *Scientific reports*, *9*(1), 2204. doi:10.1038/s41598-019-39700-6

Bolten, W. W., Glade, M. J., Raum, S., & Ritz, B. W. (2015). The safety and efficacy of an enzyme combination in managing knee osteoarthritis pain in adults: a randomized, double-blind, placebo-controlled trial. *Arthritis*, *2015*, 251521. doi:10.1155/2015/251521

Birnbaum, L.S. (2013). When environmental chemicals act like uncontrolled medicine. *Trends Endocrinol Metab*, 24:321–323. doi: 10.1016/j.tem.2012.12.005.

Bredhult, C., Bäcklin, B.M., Olovsson, M. (2007). Effects of some endocrine disruptors on the proliferation and viability of human endometrial endothelial cells in vitro. *Reprod Toxicol. 2007*, 23:550–559. doi: 10.1016/j.reprotox.2007.03.006.

Brichant, G., Patricia, N., Adelin, A., Carine, M., Foidart, J-M., & Nisolle, M. (2018). Heterogeneity of estrogen receptor α and progesterone receptor distribution in lesions of deep infiltrating endometriosis of untreated women or during exposure to various hormonal treatments. *Gynecological Endocrinology*, DOI: 10.1080/09513590.2018.1433160

Buchwald-Werner, S., Fujii, H., Reule, C., & Schoen, C. (2014). Perilla extract improves gastrointestinal discomfort in a randomized placebo controlled double blind human pilot study. *BMC complementary and alternative medicine*, 14, 173. doi:10.1186/1472-6882-14-173

Buck Louis, G.M., Peterson, C.M., Chen, Z., Croughan, M., Sundaram, R., Stanford, J., Varner, M.W., Kennedy, A., Giudice, L., Fujimoto, V.Y., Sun, L., Wang, L., Guo, Y., & Kannan, K. (2013). Bisphenol A and phthalates and endometriosis: the Endometriosis: Natural History, Diagnosis and Outcomes Study. *Fertil Steril (e1-2)*, 100:162–169. doi: 10.1016/j.fertnstert.2013.03.026.

Buck Louis, G.M., Sundaram, R., Sweeney, A.M., Schisterman, E.F., Maisog, J., & Kannan, K. (2014). Urinary bisphenol A, phthalates, and couple fecundity: the Longitudinal Investigation of Fertility and the Environment (LIFE) Study. *Fertil Steril*, 101:1359–1366. doi: 10.1016/j.fertnstert.2014.01.022.

Burney, R. O., & Giudice, L. C. (2012). Pathogenesis and Pathophysiology of Endometriosis. *Fertility and Sterility*, 98(3), 10.1016/j.fertnstert.2012.06.029. http://doi.org/10.1016/ j.fertnstert.2012.06.029

Butler, D.G. & Moseley, L. (2015). *The Explain Pain Handbook Protectometer.*

Caserta, D., Mallozzi, M., Pulcinelli, F.M., Mossa, B., & Moscarini, M. (2016). Endometriosis allergic or autoimmune disease: pathogenetic aspects–a case control study. *Clin Exp Obstet Gynecol*, 43(3), 354-7.

Cassady, B.A., Hollis, J.H., Fulford, A.D., Considine, R.V., & Mattes, R.D. (2009). Mastication of almonds: effects of lipid bioaccessibility, appetite, and hormone response. *Am J Clin Nutr*, 89(3),794-800. doi: 10.3945/ajcn.2008.26669.

Chedid, V., Dhalla, S., Clarke, J. O., Roland, B. C., Dunbar, K. B., Koh, J., ... Mullin, G. E. (2014). Herbal therapy is equivalent to rifaximin for the treatment of small intestinal bacterial overgrowth. *Global advances in health and medicine*, 3(3), 16–24. doi:10.7453/gahmj.2014.019

Chen, C., Song, X., Wei, W., Zhong, H., Dai, J., Lan, Z., ... Jia, H. (2017). The microbiota continuum along the female reproductive tract and its relation to uterine-related diseases. *Nature communications*, 8(1), 875. doi:10.1038/s41467-017-00901-0

Cramer, D.W., Goldstein, D.P., Fraer, C., et al. (1996). Vaginal agenesis (Mayer-Rokitansky-Kuster- Hauser syndrome) associated with the N314D mutation of galactose-1-phosphate uridyl trans- ferase (GALT). *Mol Hum Reprod,* 2: 145–148.

Dennis, C.H., Clohessy D.S., Stone AL, Darnall BD, & Wilson AC. (2019) Adverse Childhood Experiences in Mothers With Chronic Pain and Intergenerational Impact on Children. *J Pain*, 20(10),1209-1217. doi: 10.1016/j.jpain.2019.04.004.

Drummond, J., Ford, D., Daniel, S., & Meyerink, T. (2016). Vulvodynia and Irritable Bowel Syndrome Treated With an Elimination Diet: A Case Report. *Integrative medicine (Encinitas, Calif.)*, *15*(4), 42–47.

Drummond, J. (2018). Functional Nutrition Treatment of Vulvodynia, Irritable Bowel Syndrome, and Depression: A Case Report. *Integrative medicine (Encinitas, Calif.)*, *17*(3), 44–51.

Dun, E. C., Kho, K. A., Morozov, V. V., Kearney, S., Zurawin, J. L., & Nezhat, C. H. (2015). Endometriosis in adolescents. *JSLS : Journal of the Society of Laparoendoscopic Surgeons*, *19*(2), e2015.00019. doi:10.4293/JSLS.2015.00019

Dunselman G.A., Vermeulen, N., Becker, C., Calhaz-Jorge, C., D'Hooghe, T., De Bie, B., Heikinheimo, O., Horne, A.W., Kiesel, L., Nap, A., Prentice, A., Saridogan, E., Soriano, D., & Nelen, W. (2014). European Society of Human Reproduction and Embryology ESHRE guideline: management of women with endometriosis. *Hum Reprod*, 29(3):400–12.

Eisenber, V.E., Zoltu, M., & Soriano, D. (2012) Is there an association between autoimmunity and endometriosis? *Autoimmun Rev*, 11(11), 806-14. doi: 10.1016/j.autrev.2012.01.005.

Ek, M., Roth, B., Nilsson, P.M., & Ohlsson, B. (2018). Characteristics of endometriosis: A case-cohort study showing elevated IgG titers against the TSH receptor (TRAb) and mental comorbidity, *Eur J Obstet Gynecol Reprod Biol*, 231, 8-14. doi: 10.1016/j.ejogrb.2018.09.034.

Eskenazi, B., Mocarelli, P., Warner, M., Samuels, S., Vercellini, P., Olive, D., Needham, L.L., Patterson Jr, D.G., Brambilla, P., Gavoni, N., Casalini, S., Panazza, S., Turner, W., & Gerthoux, P.M. (2002). Serum dioxin concentrations and endometriosis: a cohort study in Seveso, Italy. *Environ Health Perspect*, 110:629–634. doi: 10.1289/ehp.02110629.

Faccin, F., Barbara, G., Saita, E., Mosconi, P., Roberto, A., Fedele, L., & Vercellini, P. (2015). Impact of endometriosis on quality of life and mental health: pelvic pain makes the difference. *J Psychosom Obstet Gynaecol*, 36(4), 135-41. doi: 10.3109/0167482X.2015.1074173.

Feliu-Soler, A., Montesinos, F., Gutiérrez-Martínez, O., Scott, W., McCracken, L. M., & Luciano, J. V. (2018). Current status of acceptance and commitment therapy for chronic pain: a narrative review. *Journal of pain research*, *11*, 2145–2159. doi:10.2147/JPR. S144631

Ferrero S1,2, Evangelisti G1,2, Barra F. (2018) Current and emerging treatment options for endometriosis, *Expert Opin Pharmacother*, 19(10):1109-1125. doi: 10.1080/14656566.2018.1494154.

Fierens, S., Mairesse, H., Heilier, J.F., De Burbure, C., Focant, J.F., Eppe, G., De Pauw, E., & Bernard, A. (2003). Dioxin/polychlorinated biphenyl body burden, diabetes and endometriosis: findings in a population-based study in Belgium. *Biomarkers*, 8,529–534. doi: 10.1080/1354750032000158420.

Fluyau, D., Revadigar, N., & Manobianco, B. E. (2018). Challenges of the pharmacological management of benzodiazepine withdrawal, dependence, and discontinuation. *Therapeutic advances in psychopharmacology*, *8*(5), 147–168. doi:10.1177/2045125317753340

Fung, J.N., & Montgomery, G.W. (2018) Genetics of endometriosis: state of the art on genetic risk factors for endometriosis. *Best Practice & Research Clinical Obstetrics & Gynaecology*, doi: 10.1016/j.bpobgyn.2018.01.012.

Giacosa, A., Guido, D., Grassi, M., Riva, A., Morazzoni, P., Bombardelli, E., ... Rondanelli, M. (2015). The Effect of Ginger (Zingiber officinalis) and Artichoke (Cynara cardunculus) Extract Supplementation on Functional Dyspepsia: A Randomised, Double-Blind, and Placebo-Controlled Clinical Trial. *Evidence-based complementary and alternative medicine: eCAM*, *2015*, 915087. doi:10.1155/2015/915087

Goetz, L. G., Mamillapalli, R., & Taylor, H. S. (2016). Low Body Mass Index in Endometriosis Is Promoted by Hepatic Metabolic Gene Dysregulation in Mice. *Biology of reproduction*, *95*(6), 115. doi:10.1095/biolreprod.116.142877

Goncalves, A.V., Barros, N.F., & Bahamondes, L. (2017). The Practice of Hatha Yoga for the Treatment of Pain Associated with Endometriosis. *J Altern Complement Med*, 23(1), 45-52. doi: 10.1089/acm.2015.0343.

Grandi, G., Barra, F., Ferrero, S., Sileo, F.G., Bertucci, E., Napolitano, A., & Facchinetti, F. (2019). Hormonal contraception in women with endometriosis: a systematic review. *Eur J Contracept Reprod Health Care*, 24(1):61-70. doi: 10.1080/13625187.2018.1550576.

Healey, M., Cheng, C., & Kaur, H. (2014). To excise or ablate endometriosis? A prospective randomized double-blinded trial after 5-year follow-up. *J Minim Invasive Gynecol*, 21(6),999–1004.

Heilier, J.F., Nackers, F., Verougstraete, V., Tonglet, R., Lison, D., & Donnez, J. (2005). Increased dioxin-like compounds in the serum of women with peritoneal endometriosis and deep endometriotic (adenomyotic) nodules. *Fertil Steril*, 84:305–312. doi: 10.1016/j.fertnstert.2005.04.001.

Hirschtritt, M. E., Delucchi, K. L., & Olfson, M. (2017). Outpatient, combined use of opioid and benzodiazepine medications in the United States, 1993-2014. *Preventive medicine reports*, 9, 49–54. doi:10.1016/j.pmedr.2017.12.010

Holoch, K.J., Savaris, R.F., Forstein, D.A., Miller, P.B., Higdon, H.L., Likes, C.E., & Lessey, B.A. (2014). Coexistence of polycystic ovary syndrome and endometriosis in women with infertility. *Pelvic Pain Disord*, 6(2), 79 - 83, DOI:10.5301/je.5000181.

Huang, P.C., Tsai, E.M., Li, W.F., Liao, P.C., Chung, M.C., Wang, Y.H., & Wang, S.L. (2010). Association between phtalate exposure and glutathione S-transferase M1 polymorphism in adenomyosis, leiomioma and endometriosis. *Hum Reprod,* 25, 986–994. doi: 10.1093/humrep/deq015.

Indiani, C.M.D.S.P., Rizzardi, K.F., Castelo, P.M., Ferraz, L.F.C., Darrieux, M, & Parisotto, T.M. (2018). Childhood Obesity and Firmicutes/Bacteroidetes Ratio in the Gut Microbiota: A Systematic Review, *Child Obes*, 14(8), 501-509. doi: 10.1089/chi.2018.0040.

Jacka, F. N., O'Neil, A., Opie, R., Itsiopoulos, C., Cotton, S., Mohebbi, M., … Berk, M. (2017). A randomised controlled trial of dietary improvement for adults with major depression (the 'SMILES' trial). *BMC medicine*, 15(1), 23. doi:10.1186/s12916-017-0791-y

Janssen, E.B., Rijkers, A.C.M., Hoppenbrouwers, K., Meuleman, K., & D'Hooghe, T.M. (2013). Prevalence of endometriosis diagnosed by laparoscopy in adolescents with dysmenorrhea or chronic pelvic pain: a systematic review. *Human Reproduction Update*, 19(5), 570–582, https://doi.org/ 10.1093/humupd/dmt016.

Kennedy, S., Bergqvist, A., Chapron, C., D'Hooghe, T., Dunselman, G., Greb, R., Hummelshoj, L., Prentice, A., & Saridogan, E. (2005) ESHRE Special Interest Group for Endometriosis and Endometrium Guideline Development Group. ESHRE guideline for the diagnosis and treatment of endometriosis. *Hum Reprod,*20(10), 2698–704.

Kim, S.H., Chun, S., Jang, J.Y., Chae, H.D., Kim, C.H., & Kang, B.M. (2011). Increased plasma levels of phthalate esters in women with advanced-stage endometriosis: a prospective case-control study. *Fertil Steril,* 95, 357–359. doi: 10.1016/j. fertnstert.2010.07.1059.

Koliada, A., Syzenko, G., Moseiko, V., Budovska, L., Puchkov, K., Perederiy, V., ... Vaiserman, A. (2017). Association between body mass index and Firmicutes/Bacteroidetes ratio in an adult Ukrainian population. *BMC microbiology, 17*(1), 120. doi:10.1186/s12866-017-1027-1

Krishnamoorthy, K. & Decherney, A.H. (2017). Genetics of Endometriosis. *Clinical Obstetrics and Gynecology,* 60(3), 531-538.

Kvaskoff, M., Han, J., Qureshi, A.A., & Missmer, S.A. (2014). Pigmentary traits, family history of melanoma and the risk of endometriosis: a cohort study of US women. *Int J Epidemiol,* 43, 255–263

Kvaskoff, M., Mu, F., Terry, K. L., Harris, H. R., Poole, E. M., Farland, L., & Missmer, S. A. (2015). Endometriosis: a high-risk population for major chronic diseases? *Human Reproduction Update*, 21(4), 500– 516. http://doi.org/10.1093/humupd/dmv013.

Lamvu, G., Soliman, A. M., Manthena, S. R., Gordon, K., Knight, J., & Taylor, H. S. (2019). Patterns of Prescription Opioid Use in Women With Endometriosis: Evaluating Prolonged Use, Daily Dose, and Concomitant Use With Benzodiazepines. *Obstetrics and gynecology, 133*(6), 1120–1130. doi:10.1097/AOG.0000000000003267

Laschke, MW & Menger, MD (2016) The gut microbiota: a puppet master in the pathogenesis of endometriosis? *American Journal of Obstetrics & Gynecology*, July, 68-70

Lazzini, S, Polinelli, W, Riva, A, Morazzoni, P & Bombardelli, E. (2016) The effect of ginger (Zingiber officinalis) and artichoke (Cynara cardunculus) extract supplementation on gastric motility: a pilot randomized study in healthy volunteers, *Eur Rev Med Pharmacol Sci*, 20(1), 146-9.

Leeners, B, Damaso, F, Ochsenbein-Kölble N, & Farquhar C (2018) The effect of pregnancy on endometriosis-facts or fiction? *Hum Reprod Update,* Feb 15. doi: 10.1093/humupd/dmy004

Leone Roberti Maggiore U, Ferrero S, Mangili G, Bergamini A, Inversetti A, Giorgione V, Viganò P, & Candiani M. (2016) A systematic review on endometriosis during pregnancy: diagnosis, misdiagnosis, complications and outcomes, *Hum Reprod Update*, 22(1),70-103. doi: 10.1093/ humupd/dmv045.

Lewis, S. C., Bhattacharya, S., Wu, O., Vincent, K., Jack, S. A., Critchley, H. O., ... Horne, A. W. (2016). Gabapentin for the Management of Chronic Pelvic Pain in Women (GaPP1): A Pilot Randomised Controlled Trial. *PloS one*, *11*(4), e0153037. doi:10.1371/journal.pone.0153037

Li, X., Feng, Y., Lin, J.-F., Billig, H., & Shao, R. (2014). Endometrial progesterone resistance and PCOS. *Journal of Biomedical Science*, 21(1), 2. http://doi.org/10.1186/1423-0127-21-2

Li, J. J., Chung, J., Wang, S., Li, T. C., & Duan, H. (2018). The Investigation and Management of Adenomyosis in Women Who Wish to Improve or Preserve Fertility. *BioMed research international*, 6832685. doi:10.1155/2018/6832685.

Lin, Y. H., Chen, Y. H., Chang, H. Y., Au, H. K., Tzeng, C. R., & Huang, Y. H. (2018). Chronic Niche Inflammation in Endometriosis-Associated Infertility: Current Understanding and Future Therapeutic Strategies. *International journal of molecular sciences*, *19*(8), 2385. doi:10.3390/ijms19082385

Liu, Y., Alookaran, J. J., & Rhoads, J. M. (2018). Probiotics in Autoimmune and Inflammatory Disorders. *Nutrients*, 10(10), 1537. doi:10.3390/nu10101537

Luckow Invitti, A., Schor, E., Martins Parreira, R., Kopelman, A., Kamergorodsky, G., Gonçalves, G. A., & Batista Castello Girão, M. J. (2018). Inflammatory cytokine profile of co-cultivated primary cells from the endometrium of women with and without endometriosis. *Molecular medicine reports*, 18(2), 1287–1296. doi:10.3892/mmr.2018.9137

May KE, Villar J, Kirtley S, Kennedy SH, Becker CM. (2011) Endometrial alterations in endometriosis: a systematic review of putative biomarkers. *Hum Reprod Update*, 17(5), 637–53

Mehedintu, C., Plotogea, M. N., Ionescu, S., & Antonovici, M. (2014). Endometriosis still a challenge. *Journal of medicine and life*, *7*(3), 349–357.

Mignemi, G, Facchini, C, Raimondo, D., Montanari, G., Ferrini, G, & Seracchioli, R. (2012) A case report of nasal endometriosis in a patient affected by Behcet's disease, *J Minim Invasive Gynecol*, 19(4), 514-6. doi: 10.1016/j.jmig.2012.03.005.

Pan Q, Luo X, Toloubeydokhti T, Chegini N. (2007) The expression profile of micro-RNA in endometrium and endometriosis and the influence of ovarian steroids on their expression. *Mol Hum Reprod*, 13, 797–806.

Pankratjevaite, L., & Samiatina-Morkuniene, D. (2017). A case report of thoracic endometriosis - A rare cause of haemothorax. *International journal of surgery case reports*, *33*, 139–142. doi:10.1016/j.ijscr.2017.02.052

Parasar, P., Ozcan, P., & Terry, K. L. (2017). Endometriosis: Epidemiology, Diagnosis and Clinical Management. *Current obstetrics and gynecology reports*, 6(1), 34–41. doi:10.1007/s13669-017-0187-1

Pauwels A, Schepens PJ, D'Hooghe T, Delbeke L, Dhont M, Brouwer A, Weyler J. (2001) The risk of endometriosis and exposure to dioxins and polychlorinated bisphenyls: a case control study of infertile women. *Hum Reprod,* 16, 2050–2055. doi: 10.1093/humrep/16.10.2050.

Piazza, M. J., & Urbanetz, A. A. (2019). Environmental toxins and the impact of other endocrine disrupting chemicals in women's reproductive health. *JBRA assisted reproduction*, 23(2), 154–164. doi:10.5935/1518-0557.20190016

Pizzorno J. (2015) Conventional Laboratory Tests to Assess Toxin Burden. *Integr Med (Encinitas)*, 14(5), 8-16. PMID: 26770160; PMCID: PMC4712864.

Poole, EM, Lin, WT, Kvaskoff, M, DeVivo, I, Terry, KL, & Missmer, SA (2017) Endometriosis and risk of ovarian and endometrial cancers in a large prospective cohort of U.S. nurses, *Cancer Causes Control*, 28(5), 437-445. doi: 10.1007/s10552-017-0856-4.

Porpora MG, Medda E, Abballe A, Bolli S, De Angelis I, di Domenico A, Ferro A, Ingelido AM, Maggi A, Panici PB, De Felip E. (2009) Endometriosis and organochlorinated environmental pollutants:a case-control study on italian women of reproductive age. *Environ Health Perspect*, 117, 1070–1075. doi: 10.1289/ehp.0800273.

Ravn, S. L., Vaegter, H. B., Cardel, T., & Andersen, T. E. (2018). The role of posttraumatic stress symptoms on chronic pain outcomes in chronic pain patients referred to rehabilitation. *Journal of pain research*, 11, 527–536. doi:10.2147/JPR. S155241

Reynolds, K, Kaufman, R, Korenoski, A, Fennimore, L, Shulman, J & Lynch, M. (2019) Trends in gabapentin and baclofen exposures reported to U.S. poison centers, Clinical Toxicology, DOI: 10.1080/15563650.2019.1687902

Rier SE, Turner WE, Martin DC, Morris R, Lucier GW, Clark GC. (2001) Serum levels of TCDD and dioxine-like chemicals in Rhesus monkeys chronically exposed to dioxin: correlation of increased serum PCB levels with endometriosis. *Toxicol Sci,* 59, 147–159. doi: 10.1093/toxsci/59.1.147.

Rizk, B., Turki, R., Lotfy, H., Ranganathan, S., Zahed, H., Freeman, A. R. Malik, R. (2015). Surgery for endometriosis-associated infertility: do we exaggerate the magnitude of effect? *Facts, Views & Vision in ObGyn*, 7(2), 109–118.

Rogers PA, et al. (2009) Priorities for endometriosis research: recommendations from an international consensus workshop. *Reprod Sci,* 16(4), 335-46.

Rolla E. (2019). Endometriosis: advances and controversies in classification, pathogenesis, diagnosis, and treatment. *F1000Research*, *8*, F1000 Faculty Rev-529. doi:10.12688/f1000research.14817.1

Romani M, Pistillo MP, Banelli B. (2015) Environmental Epigenetics: Crossroad between Public Health, Lifestyle, and Cancer Prevention. *BioMed Res Int* 2015:587983. doi: 10.1155/2015/587983.

Saha R, Pettersson HJ, Svedberg P, Olovsson M, Bergqvist A, Marions L, et al. (2015) Heritability of endometriosis. *Fertil Steril,* 104(4), 947-52.

Samulowitz, A., Gremyr, I., Eriksson, E., & Hensing, G. (2018). "Brave Men" and "Emotional Women": A Theory-Guided Literature Review on Gender Bias in Health Care and Gendered Norms towards Patients with Chronic Pain. *Pain research & management*, 6358624. doi:10.1155/2018/6358624

Simmen, R., & Kelley, A. S. (2018). Seeing red: diet and endometriosis risk. *Annals of translational medicine*, 6(Suppl 2), S119. doi:10.21037/atm.2018.12.14

Simsa P, Mihalyi A, Schoeters G, Koppen G, Kyama CM, Den Hond EM, Fülöp V, D'Hooghe TM. (2010) Increased exposure to dioxine-likecompounds is associated with endometriosis in a case-control study in women. *Reprod Biomed Online,* 20, 681–688. doi: 10.1016/j.rbmo.2010.01.018.

Somigliana E, Vigano P, Parazzini F, et al. (2006) Association between endometriosis and cancer: a comprehensive review and a critical analysis of clinical and epidemiological evidence. *Gynecol Oncol*, 101:331–41.

Stenberg G., Fjellman-Wiklund, A., & Ahlgren, C. (2014). 'I am afraid to make the damage worse'–fear of engaging in physical activity among patients with neck or back pain–a gender perspective. *Scandinavian Journal of Caring Sciences*, 28(1), 146–154. doi: 10.1111/scs.12043

Stephansson, O., Falconer, H. & Ludvigsson, J.F. (2011). Risk of endometriosis in 11,000 women with celiac disease. *Hum Reprod*, 26(10), 2896-901. doi: 10.1093/humrep/der263.

Teng, S.W., Horng, H.C., Ho, C.H., Yen, M.S., Chao, H.T., & Wang, P.H., et al. (2016). Women with endometriosis have higher comorbidities: analysis of domestic data in Taiwan. *J Chin Med Assoc,* 79, 577–582.

Timmons, J. (2018). Ovarian Cancer: Facts, Statistics, and You, Healthline, https://www.healthline.com/health/cancer/ovari-an-cancer-facts-statistics-infographic#1 accessed July 24, 2019.

Treloar, S.A., O'Connor, D.T., O'Connor, V.M., & Martin, N.G. (1999). Genetic influences on endometriosis in an Australian twin sample. *Fertil Steril,* 71(4), 701-10.

Tu, K., As-Sanie, S., Soliman, A.M., Chiuve, S., Cross, S., Eichner, S., Flores, O.A., Horne, A., Schneider, B., & Missmer, S. (2019). Impact of Endometriosis on Women's Life Decisions and Goal Attainment: Survey Results, Presented at The Annual Meeting of The International Pelvic Pain Society, Toronto, CA.

Upson, K., Sathyanarayana, S., De Roos, A.J., Thompson, M.L., Scholes, D., Dills, R., & Holt, V.L. (2013). Phthalates and risk of endometriosis. *Environ Res* 126, 91–97. doi: 10.1016/j.envres.2013.07.003.

Vannuccini, S., Lazzeri, L., Orlandi, C., Morgante, G., Bifulco, G., Fagiolini, A., & Petraglia, F. (2017). Mental health, pain symptoms and systemic comorbidities in women with endometriosis: a cross-sectional study. *J Psychosom Obstet Gynaecol*, 13, 1-6. doi: 10.1080/0167482X.2017.1386171.

Vasquez, A. (2017). *Inflammation Mastery, 4th Edition*, https://www.academia.edu/26378508/Inflammation_Mastery_4th_Edi-tion accessed on July 24, 2019.

Vigano, D., Zara, F., & Usai, P. (2018). Irritable bowel syndrome and endometriosis: New insights for old diseases. *Dig Liver Dis*, 50(3), 213-219. doi: 10.1016/j.dld.2017.12.017.

Vodolazkaia, A., El-Aalamat, Y., Popovic, D., Mihalyi, A., Bossuyt, X., Kyama, C.M., Fassbender, A., Bokor, A., Schols, D., Huskens, D., Meuleman, C., Peeraer, K., Tomassetti, C., Gevaert, O., Waelkens, E., Kasran, A., De Moor, B., D'Hooghe, T.M. (2012). Evaluation of a panel of 28 biomarkers for the non-invasive diagnosis of endometriosis. *Hum Reprod,* 27(9), 2698–711.

Wei, J.J., William, J., & Bulun, S. (2011). Endometriosis and Ovarian Cancer: A Review of Clinical, Pathologic, and Molecular Aspects. *International Journal of Gynecological Pathology : Official Journal of the International Society of Gynecological Pathologists*, 30(6), 553–568. http:// doi.org/10.1097/PGP.0b013e31821f4b85

Werner, A., Steihaug, S., & Malterud, K. (2003). Encountering the continuing challenges for women with chronic pain: recovery through recognition. *Qualitative Health Research*, 13(4), 491–509. doi: 10.1177/1049732302250755.

Acknowledgments

Thank you to every one of my patients, clients, colleagues, and students. I learn from you every day and am constantly inspired by your dedication and courage.

Thanks to every endometriosis researcher. Your tireless work is essential for those of us on the front lines to keep doing our work.

A special thank you to Heather Pierce Giannone and Mallory Leone for their assistance with recipe development.

Thanks Mom and Dad for giving me the gift of an amazing education and constantly encouraging me. The foundation of those gifts gives me the ability to be innovative and creative to find solutions to the devastating disease of endometriosis.

Thanks, Mark, for your constant love and support! And thanks Claire and Kate for keeping life amazing and fun! We have the best family ever and you're the reason for everything I do.

Thank You Page

Thank you so much for reading *Outsmart Endometriosis*. I hope that you enjoyed learning about this complete, integrative method for managing your endometriosis symptoms so you can grab hold of career and life opportunities as they come to you! I hope that you feel more empowered and have a clearer plan for your healing journey and career path.

As my gift to you, get your complete bonus package here: **http://outsmartendo.com/**

Your complete bonus package includes your Web of Support Guide, recommended lab testing and supplement resources, a full color printable recipe guide, sexual health resources, and much more!

Website: https://integrativewomenshealthinstitute.com/
Email: jessica@integrativewomenshealthinstitute.com
Facebook: https://www.facebook.com/IntegrativePelvicHealth/
Instagram: https://www.instagram.com/integrativewomenshealth/
Twitter: https://twitter.com/jessrdrummond
LinkedIn: https://www.linkedin.com/in/jessicarobilottodrummond/

About the Author

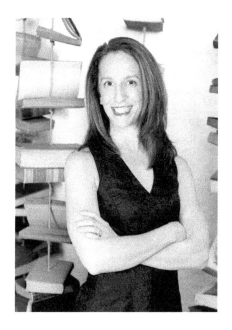

Dr. Jessica Drummond, DCN, CNS, PT, NBC-HWC is the founder and CEO of The Integrative Women's Health Institute and the author of *Outsmart Endometriosis*. She is passionate about caring for and empowering people who struggle with women's and pelvic health concerns. She is equally passionate about educating and supporting clinicians and wellness professionals in confidently and safely using integrative tools to transform women's and pelvic healthcare.

Dr. Drummond has two decades of clinical experience as a licensed physical therapist, licensed clinical nutritionist, and board-certified health coach working with women with pelvic pain, including endometriosis, vulvodynia, and bladder pain syndrome. She brings a unique conservative and integrative approach to supporting women to overcome hormonal imbalances and chronic pain conditions. She is a sought-after international speaker on topics such as integrative pelvic pain management, natural fertility options, optimal hormone health, and female athlete nutrition.

She loves farmers' markets, art museums, eating great food, and having girls' movie nights with her daughters. She lives and works from her home and offices in Fairfield, Connecticut, and Houston, Texas, reaching thousands of clients and professional students in over sixty countries through her virtual practice and educational programs.

Dr. Drummond was educated at the University of Virginia, Emory University, Duke Integrative Medicine, and Maryland University of Integrative Health.

CPSIA information can be obtained
at www.ICGtesting.com
Printed in the USA
JSHW040849160121
10868JS00001B/1